ESSENTIAL

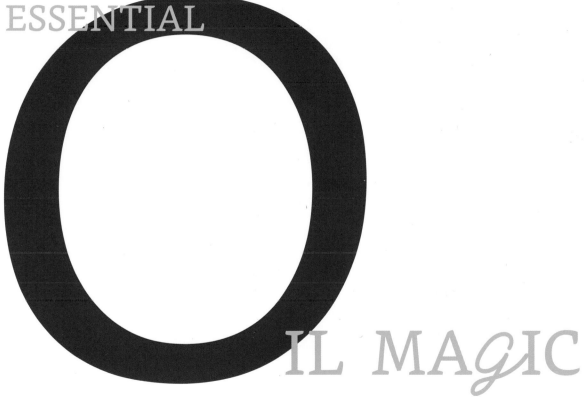

OIL MAGIC

1st Edition

Essential Oil Magic
Easy-to-Use Guidebook + Tearaway Protocols

1st Edition August 2017

ISBN: 978-0-9993689-0-9

Published by:

Oil Magic Publishing
Pleasant Grove, Utah
contact@oilmagicguide.com

About this book

This book is for the lovers of doing things naturally. You can create magic when you have the right ingredients, and essential oils seem almost just like that: magical.

Use this guide as your first go-to. Turn to nature as your first resort, and remember that you also have the power of western medicine when needed.

When you make a habit of using natural remedies like essential oils, you learn that you have the ability to create the wellness you want. Your oils are a treasure trove. They're versatile, they rarely produce side-effects, and they're friendly to your pocket book when you compare them to doctor visits and medication costs.

Enjoy all the things your oils can do for you. Enjoy the aromas, and have fun blending oils to make your own aromas. Try creative DIY projects, or even put a drop of oil in your cooking or baking.

Most importantly, see what happens to your confidence as you learn to trust nature and yourself with your family's wellness.

Use the Ailments section as a quick reference guide to find natural remedies for your health concerns. Discover the top uses of popular essential oils in the Single Oils and Oil Blends sections. Use the Protocols section to get serious results. And share the tearaway protocols in Protocols for Sharing with friends!

Have fun creating your magic.

Table of *Contents*

Section 1

Simplified Usage Guide

Uses

1 ^A
Aromatic

Diffuse
Put 4-8 drops in a diffuser to spread the oil throughout the room.

From Hands
Inhale a couple drops from cupped hands.

From Bottle
Enjoy the aroma directly from the bottle.

2 ^T
Topical

Neat
Apply certain oils directly to skin without dilution.

Dilute
Dilute with Fractionated Coconut Oil or other carrier oil/lotion as needed.

Roller Bottle
Put 10-20 drops in a roller bottle. Fill the rest with Fractionated Coconut Oil.

3 ^I
Internal

Veggie Capsule
Put oils in an empty veggie cap, and take with water.

Drink with Water
Drink 1-2 drops with water (for oils with a friendly taste).

Most brands of oils are not safe for internal use. Be sure yours has undergone strict gas chromatography and mass spectrometry to ensure purity and chemical soundness.

Safety

Children

Essential oils are safe to use with children in smaller amounts. The smaller the child, the less essential oil needed. Use this chart as a general guideline for use with children.

Age	Topical Dilution Ratio*	Internal Use
Birth - 12 months	1:30	1 drop (3-12 drops in 12 hours)
1-5 years	1:20	1 drop (3-12 drops in 12 hours)
6-11 years	1:15	1-2 drops (3-12 drops in 12 hours)

*essential oil : carrier oil

Medication

Always consult with a physician if you have questions about using an essential oil with a medication. While certain foods may interact with medications, essential oils frequently require less restraint because of the chemical makeup of the oil vs. the food.

Pregnancy

Essential oils are wonderful for pregnancy support. Oils can be used in smaller doses, and certain oils should be avoided: Birch[ATI], Cassia[TI], Cinnamon[TI], Cypress[I], Eucalyptus[I], Rosemary[ATI], Thyme[ATI], Wintergreen[TI].

Sensitive Skin

Dilute as needed for sensitive skin. Apply to the bottoms of feet to avoid sensitivity.

Preference & Purpose

Remember that while essential oils have a most useful purpose, you should also enjoy what you use! Enjoying the use of oils makes it easier to create lifestyle habits with them.

If you love the smell of an essential oil, use away! If you don't love the smell, try an application method that limits exposure to the fragrance (like in a veggie cap or on the bottoms of feet), or look for a different oil that has similar properties.

Blending

Remember that you can't break your oils. If you experiment with blending, but don't succeed, try again. You'll learn the smells that resonate best with you.

Sometimes you'll find yourself in need of an oil you may not love. Try combining it with another oil to create a fragrance you enjoy.

Here are some blending tips:

• Pay attention to low, mid, and high notes in your oils for a well-rounded fragrance. (e.g. Vetiver is a low note, Lavender is a mid note, and Lemon is a high note.)

• Add FCO to your blends to help the fragrance last longer.

• When layering oils topically (using multiple oils one on top of the other), the oils on top will generally smell the strongest.

How much oil should I use?

Discover what works best for your body. Take heed of the safety warnings for each oil in this book. *Remember - small amounts more frequently tend to produce the best results.*

Section 2

Ailments &
Conditions

Ailments

Acid Reflux A T I

Take 1-2 drops internally or apply to stomach area as needed.

Peppermint T I
Digestive Blend T I
Ginger T I
Dill T I
Digestion Tablets I
Protocol on pg. 164

ADD & ADHD A T I

Apply a few drops on forehead and back of neck; inhale a few drops from cupped hands.

Focus Blend A T
Reassuring Blend A T
Vetiver A T I
Frankincense A T I
Grounding Blend A T
Protocol on pg. 153

Aging A T I

Apply 1-3 drops to target areas. Combine 2-8 drops with facial lotion or carrier oil and apply after cleansing.

Anti-Aging Blend T
Frankincense T I
Cedarwood T
Sandalwood T I
Vitality Trio I

Allergies (seasonal) A T I

Apply to back of neck, under nose, on bridge of nose, or chest as needed. Take a few drops internally or diffuse into the air and inhale.

Lavender A T I
Peppermint A T I
Respiratory Blend A T
Detoxification Blend A T I
Cleansing Blend A T
Protocol on pg. 154

Acne/Blemishes A T I

Apply a drop topically to affected areas. Add 2-3 drops to lotion and apply after cleansing routine.

Melaleuca T I
Lavender T I
Skin Clearing Blend T
Juniper Berry T I
Neroli T I
Protocol on pg. 152

Adrenal Fatigue A T I

Massage 1-3 drops onto lower back over adrenals, or inhale from cupped hands. Take 1-3 drops internally as needed.

Basil A T I
Juniper Berry A T I
Rosemary A T I
Geranium A T I
Ylang Ylang A T I
Protocol on pg. 153

Alertness A T I

Apply to forehead, temples, or base of skull as needed; inhale from cupped hands.

Focus Blend A T
Massage Blend A T
Basil A T I
Rosemary A T I
Peppermint A T I

Alzheimer's A T I

Massage 1-2 drops rosemary into scalp once daily. Take 1-2 drops internally 1-2 times daily. Regular supplementation for ongoing support.

Frankincense A T I
Rosemary A T I
Cellular Complex A T I
Clove A T I
Vitality Trio I
Protocol on pg. 155

12

Anemia

Apply 1-3 drops to bottoms of feet and inside of wrists; take a few drops internally; or inhale from cupped hands periodically.

Protective Blend [T][I]
Basil [T][I]
Lemon [T][I]
Lavender [T][I]
Vitality Trio [I]

Anger

Apply 1-3 drops to temples and/or chest; inhale a few drops from cupped hands as needed.

Restful Blend [A][T]
Grounding Blend [A][T]
Reassuring Blend [A][T]
Renewing Blend [A][T]
Melissa [A][T][I]

Ankle Swelling

Massage ankles with 2-4 drops, diluted with carrier oil if desired.

Juniper Berry [T]
Cypress [T]
Lemongrass [T]
Soothing Blend [T]
Tension Blend [T]

Anorexia

Apply 1-3 drops to stomach area or inhale from cupped hands as needed.

Grapefruit [A][T][I]
Metabolic Blend [A][T][I]
Invigorating Blend [A][T]
Joyful Blend [A][T]
Uplifting Blend [A][T]

Anxiety

Apply 1-3 drops to bottoms of feet, chest, or temples, or inhale from cupped hands as needed.

Grounding Blend [A][T]
Vetiver [A][T][I]
Reassuring Blend [A][T]
Neroli [A][T][I]
Cedarwood [A][T]
Protocol on pg. 155

Apathy

Apply 1-3 drops to bottoms of feet, chest, or temples, or inhale from cupped hands as needed.

Patchouli [A][T][I]
Neroli [A][T][I]
Rose [A][T]
Jasmine [A][T]
Renewing Blend [A][T]

Appetite Suppressant

Apply 1-3 drops to stomach, chest, bottoms of feet, or inside of wrists or take 1-2 drops internally.

Metabolic Blend [A][T][I]
Peppermint [A][T][I]
Grapefruit [A][T][I]
Ginger [A][T][I]
Wild Orange [A][T][I]

Arthritic Pain

Apply 1-3 drops and massage into affected areas with lotion or carrier oil as needed.

Soothing Blend [T]
Copaiba [T][I]
Wintergreen [T]
Massage Blend [T]
Polyphenol Complex [I]
Protocol on pg. 155

Asthma

Apply 1-3 drops topically to chest, neck, under nose, and on bridge of nose, or inhale from cupped as needed.

Respiratory Blend[AT]
Eucalyptus[AT]
Rosemary[AT]
Roman Chamomile[AT]
Bergamot[AT]
Protocol on pg. 156

Athlete's Foot

Apply 1-3 drops to area between toes and around toenails 2-3 times daily. Take 1-3 drops internally of melaleuca or oregano once a day.

Melaleuca[TI]
Oregano[TI]
Skin Clearing Blend[T]
Cardamom[T]
Cleansing Blend[T]

Autism/Asperger's

Apply 1-3 drops to bottoms of feet and back of neck. Take 1-3 drops internally of cilantro or cellular complex blend 1-2 times daily.

Frankincense[ATI]
Focus Blend[AT]
Geranium[ATI]
Cilantro[ATI]
Cellular Complex[ATI]
Protocol on pg. 156

Autoimmune Issues

Apply 1-3 drops to stomach, chest, bottoms of feet, or inside of wrists when applicable. Take 1-3 drops internally daily for added support.

Cellular Complex[ATI]
Detoxification Blend[ATI]
Frankincense[ATI]
Ginger[ATI]
Vitality Trio[I]

Autointoxication

Apply 1-3 drops to stomach, chest, bottoms of feet, or inside of wrists. Take 1-3 drops internally 2-3 times daily for additional support.

Detoxification Blend[TI]
Cilantro[TI]
Thyme[TI]
Oregano[TI]
Detox Herbal Complex[I]

Back Pain

Apply 1-3 drops and massage into affected areas as needed. Use a carrier oil or lotion for increased efficacy. Take 2 capsules of Polyphenol Complex 2-3 times daily.

Soothing Blend[AT]
Massage Blend[AT]
Peppermint[ATI]
Lemongrass[ATI]
Polyphenol Complex[I]
Protocol on pg. 156

Bacterial Infection

Apply 1-3 drops with a carrier oil to the affected areas as needed. Take 1-3 drops internally every 2-3 hours for systemic and/or internal infections.

Thyme[TI]
Oregano[TI]
Protective Blend[TI]
Litsea[TI]
Arborvitae[T]

Balance Problems

Apply 1-3 drops topically to forehead, temples, back of neck, and behind the ears or inhale from cupped hands. Take 1-3 drops internally of Ginger as needed.

Ginger[ATI]
Peppermint[ATI]
Basil[ATI]
Cypress[AT]
Grounding Blend[AT]

Bed Wetting

Massage 1-3 drops over urinary areas of bladder and kidneys before bedtime as needed.

Cypress ᴬ ᵀ
Black Pepper ᴬ ᵀ ᴵ
Ylang Ylang ᴬ ᵀ ᴵ
Lemongrass ᴬ ᵀ ᴵ
Roman Chamomile ᴬ ᵀ ᴵ

Bee Sting

Apply 1-2 drops topically to sting or bite several times daily until symptoms cease.

Cleansing Blend ᵀ
Roman Chamomile ᵀ
Basil ᵀ
Lemongrass ᵀ
Lavender ᵀ

Bell's Palsy

Take 1-3 drops internally every 2-3 hours as desired.

Clove ᵀ ᴵ
Melissa ᵀ ᴵ
Frankincense ᵀ ᴵ
Thyme ᵀ ᴵ
Vitality Trio ᴵ

Bipolar Disorder

Apply 1-3 drops to bottoms of feet, chest, or temples, or inhale from cupped hands as needed.

Reassuring Blend ᴬ ᵀ
Frankincense ᴬ ᵀ ᴵ
Vetiver ᴬ ᵀ ᴵ
Neroli ᴬ ᵀ ᴵ
Vitality Trio ᴵ

Bladder Control

Apply 1-3 drops topically to urinary areas of bladder and kidneys as needed. Add 1-2 drops to drinking water if desired.

Rosemary ᴬ ᵀ ᴵ
Juniper Berry ᴬ ᵀ ᴵ
Cypress ᴬ ᵀ
Lavender ᴬ ᵀ ᴵ
Sandalwood ᴬ ᵀ ᴵ

Bleeding

Apply a drop topically to affected area as needed.

Helichrysum ᵀ
Myrrh ᵀ
Geranium ᵀ
Lemon ᵀ
Melaleuca ᵀ

Blisters on Feet

Apply a few drops topically to affected area.

Frankincense ᵀ
Patchouli ᵀ
Melaleuca ᵀ
Lavender ᵀ
Myrrh ᵀ

Bloating

Apply 1-3 drops to stomach, rubbing in a clockwise direction. Take 1-3 drops internally internally as needed.

Fennel ᵀ ᴵ
Digestive Blend ᵀ ᴵ
Cilantro ᵀ ᴵ
Dill ᵀ ᴵ
Peppermint ᵀ ᴵ

Protocol on pg. 163

Blood Clotting

Apply 1-3 drops to affected area or ingest a few drops internally as needed.

Clove ᵀ ᴵ
Fennel ᵀ ᴵ
Marjoram ᵀ ᴵ
Basil ᵀ ᴵ
Wintergreen ᵀ ᴵ

Blood Pressure (high)

Apply 1-3 drops to stomach, chest, bottoms of feet, or inside of wrists, or take 1-3 drops internally as needed.

Basil ᴬ ᵀ ᴵ
Marjoram ᴬ ᵀ ᴵ
Lemon ᴬ ᵀ ᴵ
Cypress ᴬ ᵀ
Ylang Ylang ᴬ ᵀ ᴵ
Protocol on pg. 157

Blood Pressure (low)

Apply 1-3 drops to stomach, chest, bottoms of feet, or inside of wrists, or ingest a few drops as needed.

Basil ᵀ ᴵ
Helichrysum ᵀ ᴵ
Cardamom ᵀ ᴵ
Cypress ᵀ
Vitality Trio ᴵ

Blood Sugar (low)

Apply 1-3 drops to stomach, chest, bottoms of feet, or inside of wrists, or take 1-3 drops internally as needed.

Coriander ᵀ ᴵ
Fennel ᵀ ᴵ
Cassia ᵀ ᴵ
Wild Orange ᵀ ᴵ
Vitality Trio ᴵ

Blurred Vision

Mix desired oils in a roller bottle with carrier oil and carefully apply around eyes 2-4 times daily. Avoid eyes.

Clary Sage ᵀ
Lemongrass ᵀ
Helichrysum ᵀ
Cellular Complex ᵀ
Anti-Aging Blend ᵀ

Body Odor

Take 1-3 drops of Cilantro, Detoxification Blend, or Dill at least once daily. Apply 1-3 drops on bottoms of feet or underarms.

Cilantro ᵀ ᴵ
Detoxification Blend ᵀ ᴵ
Arborvitae ᵀ
Dill ᵀ ᴵ
Petitgrain ᵀ ᴵ
Protocol on pg. 161

Boils

Apply 1-3 drops topically to affected areas several times daily.

Skin Clearing Blend ᵀ
Melaleuca ᵀ
Lavender ᵀ
Myrrh ᵀ
Bergamot ᵀ

Bone Pain/Break

Apply 1-3 drops topically to affected areas as needed. Massage with lotion or carrier oil to improve efficacy.

Soothing Blend ᵀ
Wintergreen ᵀ
Birch ᵀ
Helichrysum ᵀ ᴵ
Bone Nutrient Complex ᴵ

Brain Fog

Apply 1-3 drops to forehead, temples, back of neck, and behind ears or inhale from cupped hands as needed.

Peppermint ᴬᵀᴵ
Encouraging Blend ᴬᵀ
Focus Blend ᴬᵀ
Basil ᴬᵀᴵ
Vitality Trio ᴵ

Brain Injury

Apply a few drops topically to forehead, temples, base of skull, and behind the ears or diffuse into the air and inhale. Take a few drops internally as needed.

Frankincense ᴬᵀᴵ
Cellular Complex ᴬᵀᴵ
Grounding Blend ᴬᵀ
Sandalwood ᴬᵀᴵ
Vitality Trio ᴵ

Breastfeeding
(increase milk)

Massage 1-3 drops with carrier oil over breasts and apply to bottoms of feet or take internally when needed.

Fennel ᵀᴵ
Clary Sage ᵀᴵ
Basil ᵀᴵ
Dill ᵀᴵ
Bone Nutrient Complex ᴵ
Protocol on pg. 168

Brittle Nails

Apply 1-2 drops to nail bed once daily. Use supplements consistently for long-term benefits.

Arborvitae ᵀ
Fennel ᵀᴵ
Frankincense ᵀᴵ
Bone Nutrient Complex ᴵ
Vitality Trio ᴵ

Bronchitis

Apply 1-3 drops to chest and neck area, gargle hourly, or inhale from cupped hands as needed.

Respiratory Blend ᴬᵀ
Cardamom ᴬᵀᴵ
Black Pepper ᴬᵀᴵ
Roman Chamomile ᴬᵀᴵ
Bergamot ᴬᵀᴵ
Protocol on pg. 157

Bruising

Apply 1-3 drops to bruise area. Use carrier oil if desired. Reapply 2-4 times daily.

Helichrysum ᵀ
Geranium ᵀ
Cypress ᵀ
Soothing Blend ᵀ
Tension Blend ᵀ

Bunions

Apply 1-3 drops with carrier oil to affected area as needed.

Copaiba ᵀ
Lemon ᵀ
Soothing Blend ᵀ
Ginger ᵀ
Cypress ᵀ

Burns

Apply 1-3 drops to affected area hourly or as needed. For more severe, mix 2-8 drops with 4 oz witch hazel and apply as needed.

Lavender ᵀ
Melaleuca ᵀ
Helichrysum ᵀ
Anti-Aging Blend ᵀ
Cedarwood ᵀ

Cancer

Take 1-3 drops internally at least twice daily. Supplement for added support

Cellular Complex ᵀ ᴵ
Frankincense ᵀ ᴵ
Sandalwood ᵀ ᴵ
Patchouli ᵀ ᴵ
Vitality Trio ᴵ
Protocol on pg. 158

Canker Sores

Apply a drop (dilute with carrier oil) directly to canker sore or gargle several times daily until sore is gone. Also apply oil over sore outside of mouth.

Melaleuca ᵀ ᴵ
Oregano ᵀ ᴵ
Protective Blend ᵀ ᴵ
Melissa ᵀ ᴵ
Frankincense ᵀ ᴵ
Protocol on pg. 158

Carpal Tunnel

Apply 1-3 drops to affected area several times daily. Massage with carrier oil or lotion for improved efficacy.

Soothing Blend ᴬ ᵀ
Wintergreen ᴬ ᵀ
Lemongrass ᴬ ᵀ ᴵ
Marjoram ᴬ ᵀ ᴵ
Thyme ᴬ ᵀ ᴵ

Cavities

Apply 1-2 drops directly on tooth. Dilute with carrier oil if necessary.

Clove ᵀ ᴵ
Protective Blend ᵀ ᴵ
Melaleuca ᵀ ᴵ
Bone Nutrient Complex ᴵ
Vitality Trio ᴵ

Candida

Apply 1-3 drops over affected area or take 1-3 drops internally at least twice daily until symptoms subside.

Thyme ᵀ ᴵ
Oregano ᵀ ᴵ
Melaleuca ᵀ ᴵ
Spikenard ᵀ ᴵ
Cellular Complex ᵀ ᴵ
Protocol on pg. 158

Cardiovascular Disease

Apply 1-3 drops to chest or take 1-3 drops internally as needed.

Cellular Complex ᵀ ᴵ
Black Pepper ᵀ ᴵ
Geranium ᵀ ᴵ
Coriander ᵀ ᴵ
Cypress ᵀ ᴵ

Cartilage Injury

Apply 1-3 drops to affected area several times daily. Massage with carrier oil or lotion for improved efficacy.

Soothing Blend ᴬ ᵀ
Lemongrass ᴬ ᵀ ᴵ
Helichrysum ᴬ ᵀ ᴵ
Frankincense ᴬ ᵀ ᴵ
Copaiba ᴬ ᵀ ᴵ

Cellulite (Fat Deposits)

Massage 4-8 drops onto target areas daily, especially before exercising. Add to drinking water and consume throughout the day.

Metabolic Blend ᵀ ᴵ
Grapefruit ᵀ ᴵ
Lemon ᵀ ᴵ
Lemongrass ᵀ ᴵ
Eucalyptus ᵀ
Protocol on pg. 173

Chapped Skin

Apply a drop or two to affected area as often as needed. Use a carrier oil to increase efficacy.

Myrrh [T]
Roman Chamomile [T]
Anti-Aging Blend [T]
Cedarwood [T]
Frankincense [T]

Charley Horse

Massage 1-3 drops on area of concern. Use a carrier oil or lotion for improved efficacy.

Massage Blend [A T]
Soothing Blend [A T]
Marjoram [A T I]
Black Pepper [A T I]
Bergamot [A T I]

Chest Pain

Apply 1-3 drops topically to chest or ingest at least twice daily.

Protective Blend [A T I]
Cellular Complex [A T I]
Rosemary [A T I]
Wild Orange [A T I]
Marjoram [A T I]

Chicken Pox

Dilute 2-4 drops with a carrier oil and dab lightly on spots a couple times a day or ingest for immune support.

Cellular Complex [T I]
Thyme [T I]
Melaleuca [T I]
Lavender [T I]
Skin Clearing Blend [T]

Chiggers

Dilute 2-4 drops with a carrier oil and dab lightly on bites a couple times a day.

Outdoor Blend [A T]
Lemongrass [A T]
Melaleuca [A T]
Detoxification Blend [A T]
Arborvitae [A T]

Cholesterol (high)

Apply 1-3 drops to chest area, bottoms of feet, or inside of wrists; take 2-4 drops internally once daily.

Metabolic Blend [A T I]
Lavender [A T I]
Cypress [A T]
Rosemary [A T I]
Vitality Trio [I]
Protocol on pg. 159

Chronic Fatigue

Apply 2-4 drops to chest area, bottoms of feet, or inside of wrists; inhale 1-3 drops from cupped hands; supplement regularly for long-term benefits.

Encouraging Blend [A T]
Peppermint [A T I]
Basil [A T I]
Energy & Stamina [I]
Vitality Trio [I]
Protocol on pg. 163

Chronic Pain

Apply 1-3 drops to affected areas as needed, using carrier oil for improved efficacy; supplement regularly for long-term care.

Soothing Blend [A T]
Birch [A T]
Lemongrass [A T I]
Polyphenol Complex [I]
Vitality Trio [I]

Ailments

Circulation (poor)
Apply 1-3 drops to bottoms of feet; take 1-3 drops internally twice daily, or as needed.

Cypress^T
Ginger^{TI}
Black Pepper^{TI}
Basil^{TI}
Energy & Stamina^I

Cold (common)
Take 1-3 drops internally 3-6 times until symptoms subside; supplement regularly for long-term benefits.

Oregano^{ATI}
Thyme^{ATI}
Protective Blend^{ATI}
Melissa^{ATI}
Vitality Trio^I
Protocol on pg. 160

Cold Extremities
Apply 1-3 drops to bottoms of feet, chest area, and inside of wrists; take 1-2 drops internally daily as needed.

Cinnamon^{TI}
Black Pepper^{TI}
Protective Blend^{TI}
Cypress^T
Energy & Stamina^I

Cold Sores
Dilute with carrier oil and apply a drop to affected area as needed.

Clove^{TI}
Protective Blend^{TI}
Melaleuca^{TI}
Melissa^{TI}
Frankincense^{TI}
Protocol on pg. 160

Colic
Dilute 1-2 drops with a carrier oil and apply topically to stomach and back before baby goes to sleep.

Dill^T
Marjoram^T
Bergamot^T
Coriander^T
Roman Chamomile^T

Concussion
Apply 2-4 drops to forehead, temples, base of skull, and behind the ears; inhale 1-3 drops from cupped hands; take 1-3 drops internally for a few days.

Frankincense^{ATI}
Bergamot^{ATI}
Cypress^{AT}
Copaiba^{ATI}
Rosemary^{ATI}

Congestion
Apply 1-3 drops to back of neck, under nose, on bridge of nose, or chest; inhale 1-3 drops from cupped hands as needed.

Peppermint^{ATI}
Fennel^{ATI}
Eucalyptus^{AT}
Digestion Blend^{ATI}
Siberian Fir^{ATI}

Constipation
Massage 1-3 drops diluted over abdomen clockwise. Repeat as desired every 5-10 minutes until condition improves. Take 1-2 drops internally for additional support.

Digestion Blend^{TI}
Ginger^{TI}
Lemongrass^{TI}
Cilantro^{TI}
Fennel^{TI}
Protocol on pg. 163

20

Cortisol (heightened)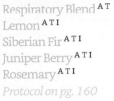

Apply 1-3 drops to back of neck, under nose, on bridge of nose, or chest as needed;. take 1-2 drops internally; inhale from cupped hands.

Ylang Ylang ᴬᵀ ᴵ
Lavender ᴬᵀ ᴵ
Clove ᴬᵀ ᴵ
Rosemary ᴬᵀ ᴵ
Coriander ᴬᵀ ᴵ
Protocol on pg. 171

Cough

Apply 1-3 drops to chest, back of neck, under nose, or on bridge of nose, as needed; inhale from cupped hands.

Respiratory Blend ᴬᵀ
Lemon ᴬᵀ ᴵ
Siberian Fir ᴬᵀ ᴵ
Juniper Berry ᴬᵀ ᴵ
Rosemary ᴬᵀ ᴵ
Protocol on pg. 160

Cramps

Massage 1-3 drops into affected areas as needed. Use with carrier oil to improve efficacy.

Soothing Blend ᴬᵀ
Arborvitae ᴬᵀ
Cypress ᴬᵀ
Women's Monthly ᴬᵀ
Massage Blend ᴬᵀ

Croup

Dilute with carrier oil and apply 1-3 drops to baby's chest and back as needed; diffuse.

Arborvitae ᴬᵀ
Lemon ᴬᵀ
Respiratory Blend ᴬᵀ
Sandalwood ᴬᵀ
Wild Orange ᴬᵀ

Crying

Apply 1-2 drops to front of shirt or sleeve, or diffuse.

Lavender ᴬᵀ
Wild Orange ᴬᵀ
Reassuring Blend ᴬᵀ
Roman Chamomile ᴬᵀ
Restful Blend ᴬᵀ

Cuts

Dilute 1-2 drops with a carrier oil and apply to affected area a couple times daily.

Lavender ᵀ
Myrrh ᵀ
Melaleuca ᵀ
Helichrysum ᵀ
Cedarwood ᵀ

Cystic Fibrosis

Apply 1-3 drops to chest and under nose; inhale from cupped hands as needed.

Sandalwood ᴬᵀ ᴵ
Respiratory Blend ᴬᵀ
Arborvitae ᴬᵀ
Myrrh ᴬᵀ ᴵ
Roman Chamomile ᴬᵀ ᴵ

Cysts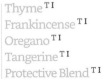

Apply 1-2 drops to affected area daily or as needed.

Thyme ᵀ ᴵ
Frankincense ᵀ ᴵ
Oregano ᵀ ᴵ
Tangerine ᵀ ᴵ
Protective Blend ᵀ ᴵ

Ailments

Dandruff

Dilute 2-6 drops in carrier oil and massage into scalp. Rinse after 60 minutes.

Cedarwood ^T
Melaleuca ^T
Rosemary ^T
Myrrh ^T
Petitgrain ^T

Dehydrated Skin

Apply 1-3 drops with carrier oil to affected area as needed. Use with lotion for improved efficacy.

Sandalwood ^T
Myrrh ^T
Anti-Aging Blend ^T
Cedarwood ^T
Coriander ^T

Dementia

Apple 1-3 drops to forehead, temples, base of skull, and behind the ears; take internally as needed; inhale from cupped hands as needed.

Frankincense ^{ATI}
Cellular Complex ^{ATI}
Clove ^{ATI}
Rosemary ^{ATI}
Peppermint ^{ATI}
Protocol on pg. 155

Depression

Apply 1-3 drops to forehead and temples; place a drop of Frankincense on thumb and press to roof of mouth; inhale from cupped hands as needed.

Joyful Blend ^{AT}
Uplifting Blend ^{AT}
Invigorating Blend ^{AT}
Frankincense ^{ATI}
Vitality Trio ^I
Protocol on pg. 161

Detoxification

Apply 3-5 drops to bottoms of feet and inside of wrists; take 1-3 drops internally a few times daily; supplement regularly for improved cleansing.

Detoxification Blend ^{TI}
Cilantro ^{TI}
Lemongrass ^{TI}
Clove ^{TI}
Detox Herbal Complex ^I
Protocol on pg. 162

Diabetes

Apply a couple drops over pancreas and bottoms of feet daily; take a few drops internally.

Cinnamon ^{TI}
Coriander ^{TI}
Juniper Berry ^{TI}
Protective Blend ^{TI}
Metabolic Blend ^{TI}
Protocol on pg. 162

Diaper Rash

Dilute 1-3 drops with carrier oil and apply to affected area several times daily until rash disappears.

Lavender ^T
Roman Chamomile ^T
Ylang Ylang ^T
Coriander ^T
Cedarwood ^T

Diarrhea

Take 2-4 drops internally; massage 1-3 drops into abdomen clockwise hourly as needed.

Digestion Blend ^{TI}
Coriander ^{TI}
Ginger ^{TI}
Patchouli ^{TI}
Spearmint ^{TI}

Diverticulitis

Take 2-4 drops internally twice daily for ongoing support; massage 1-3 drops into abdomen clockwise as needed.

Digestion Blend [TI]
Petitgrain [TI]
Basil [TI]
Cellular Complex [TI]
Digestive Enzymes [I]

Dizziness

Apply 1-3 drops to back of neck, under nose, or on temples; inhale from cupped hands; take 2-4 drops internally of Detoxification Blend as needed.

Detoxification Blend [ATI]
Grounding Blend [AT]
Cypress [AT]
Cedarwood [AT]
Arborvitae [AT]

Drug Addiction

Apply a couple drops to chest, temples, and bottoms of feet daily; inhale from cupped hands as needed.

Cassia [ATI]
Detoxification Blend [ATI]
Cleansing Blend [AT]
Black Pepper [ATI]
Renewing Blend [AT]

Dysentery

Massage 1-3 drops into abdomen; take 2-4 drops internally as needed.

Ginger [TI]
Myrrh [TI]
Oregano [TI]
Eucalyptus [T]
Siberian Fir [TI]

Dysphagia

Apply 1-3 drops to neck or ingest a few drops as needed.

Ginger [TI]
Black Pepper [TI]
Fennel [TI]
Peppermint [TI]
Spikenard [TI]

Ear Infection

Apply 1-3 drops around the opening of the ear or apply to a cotton ball and place over ear opening overnight. Do NOT use essential oils in ear. Take 2-4 drops internally.

Rosemary [T]
Basil [T]
Melaleuca [T]
Oregano [T]
Thyme [T]

Earache

Apply 1-3 drops around the opening of the ear or apply to a cotton ball and place over ear opening overnight. Do NOT use essential oils in ear.

Helichrysum [T]
Basil [T]
Ginger [T]
Petitgrain [T]
Siberian Fir [T]

Eczema

Apply 2-4 drops to affected area as needed. For improved efficacy, dilute with carrier oil.

Skin Clearing Blend [T]
Helichrysum [TI]
Cedarwood [T]
Coriander [TI]
Vitality Trio [I]
Protocol on pg. 163

Edema

Massage 1-3 drops into affected area and on bottoms of feet; ingest a couple times daily or as needed.

Juniper Berry ᵀ ᴵ
Cypress ᵀ
Lemongrass ᵀ ᴵ
Metabolic Blend ᵀ ᴵ
Grapefruit ᵀ ᴵ

Emphysema

Apply 1-3 drops to back of neck, under nose, chest, or on bridge of nose as needed; take 1-3 drops internally; inhale from cupped hands.

Respiratory Blend ᴬ ᵀ
Black Pepper ᴬ ᵀ ᴵ
Rosemary ᴬ ᵀ ᴵ
Roman Chamomile ᴬ ᵀ ᴵ
Bergamot ᴬ ᵀ ᴵ

Energy (low)

Apply 1-3 drops to bottoms of feet, under nose, on bridge of nose, or chest as needed; inhale from cupped hands as needed.

Encouraging Blend ᴬ ᵀ
Joyful Blend ᴬ ᵀ
Spearmint ᴬ ᵀ ᴵ
Energy & Stamina ᴵ
Vitality Trio ᴵ
Protocol on pg. 163

Epilepsy

Apply 1-3 drops to back of neck, under nose, or on temples or inhale from cupped hands; take 2-4 drops internally of Frankincense or Cellular Complex Blend as needed.

Frankincense ᴬ ᵀ ᴵ
Spikenard ᴬ ᵀ ᴵ
Vetiver ᴬ ᵀ ᴵ
Cellular Complex ᴬ ᵀ ᴵ
Vitality Trio ᴵ

Erectile Dysfunction

Apply 1-3 drops to temples, wrists, and back of neck as needed; inhale from cupped hands.

Cypress ᴬ ᵀ
Grounding Blend ᴬ ᵀ
Inspiring Blend ᴬ ᵀ
Sandalwood ᴬ ᵀ
Ylang Ylang ᴬ ᵀ

Estrogen Imbalance

Apply 1-3 drops to feet, abdomen, and lower back; inhale from cupped hands; ingest Clary Sage as needed.

Women's Blend ᴬ ᵀ
Basil ᴬ ᵀ ᴵ
Detoxification Blend ᴬ ᵀ ᴵ
Clary Sage ᴬ ᵀ ᴵ
Phytoestrogen Complex ᴵ

Exhaustion

Inhale 1-3 drops from cupped hands; apply a couple drops to feet and back; take 1-3 drops internally Ylang Ylang or Tangerine as needed.

Ylang Ylang ᴬ ᵀ ᴵ
Uplifting Blend ᴬ ᵀ
Encouraging Blend ᴬ ᵀ
Tangerine ᴬ ᵀ ᴵ
Peppermint ᴬ ᵀ ᴵ

Eyes (Swollen)

Apply 1-3 drops around the opening of the eye or apply to a cotton ball and place over eye. Do NOT apply into eye.

Geranium ᵀ
Siberian Fir ᵀ
Detoxification ᵀ
Patchouli ᵀ
Juniper Berry ᵀ

Fainting

Inhale 1-3 drops from cupped hands as need.

Rosemary ^{A T}
Frankincense ^{A T}
Respiratory Blend ^{A T}
Invigorating Blend ^{A T}
Eucalyptus ^{A T}

Fear

Inhale from cupped hands; apply a couple drops to feet and back.

Restful Blend ^{A T}
Wild Orange ^{A T}
Grounding Blend ^{A T}
Encouraging Blend ^{A T}
Joyful Blend ^{A T}

Fever

Apply 1-3 drops to back of neck, under nose, on bridge of nose, or chest; take 2-4 drops internally Oregano every 2-4 hours until symptoms subside.

Peppermint ^{A T I}
Oregano ^{A T I}
Eucalyptus ^{A T I}
Tension Blend ^{A T}
Soothing Blend ^{A T}

Fibrocystic Breasts

Massage 1-3 drops into breasts as needed; ingest at least twice daily.

Thyme ^{T I}
Clary Sage ^{T I}
Sandalwood ^{T I}
Geranium ^{T I}
Frankincense ^{T I}

Fibroids (Uterine)

Apply 1-3 drops to abdomen daily; take 1-3 drops internally.

Sandalwood ^{T I}
Lemongrass ^{T I}
Frankincense ^{T I}
Cellular Complex ^{T I}
Helichrysum ^{T I}

Fibromyalgia

Apply 1-3 drops to affected areas; ingest the cellular complex blend as needed; supplement regularly for long-term support.

Cellular Complex ^{A T I}
Birch ^{A T}
Wintergreen ^{A T}
Polyphenol Complex ^I
Vitality Trio ^I
Protocol on pg. 164

Flu (Influenza)

Apply 1-3 drops to chest or back over lungs; take 2-4 drops internally every 2-3 hours as desired for antiviral and immune-boosting support.

Respiratory Blend ^{A T}
Oregano ^{A T I}
Thyme ^{A T I}
Cardamom ^{A T I}
Roman Chamomile ^{A T I}
Protocol on pg. 164

Focus & Concentration

Apply 1-3 drops to forehead, temples, back of neck, and behind the ears; inhale from cupped hands as needed.

Vetiver ^{A T}
Focus Blend ^{A T}
Spearmint ^{A T}
Rosemary ^{A T}
Reassuring Blend ^{A T}
Protocol on pg. 153

Food Poisoning

Apply 1-3 drops to stomach and rub clockwise; take 2-4 drops internally every 2-4 hours as needed.

Detoxification Blend ᵀᴵ
Digestive Blend ᵀᴵ
Black Pepper ᵀᴵ
Oregano ᵀᴵ
Protective Blend ᵀᴵ

Frozen Shoulder

Apply 1-3 drops to affected area. Massage with carrier oil for improved efficacy.

Soothing Blend ᵀ
Cypress ᵀ
Siberian Fir ᵀ
Tension Blend ᵀ
Lemongrass ᵀ

Fungal Skin

Apply 1-3 drops to affected area several times daily.

Melaleuca ᵀᴵ
Arborvitae ᵀ
Neroli ᵀᴵ
Cedarwood ᵀ
Skin Clearing Blend ᵀ

Gallbladder Issues

Massage 1-3 drops over gallbladder several times daily; take 1-3 drops internally as needed.

Detoxification Blend ᵀᴵ
Basil ᵀᴵ
Metabolic Blend ᵀᴵ
Helichrysum ᵀᴵ
Tangerine ᵀᴵ

Gallbladder Stones

Apply 1-3 drops over gallbladder several times daily; take 1-3 drops internally as needed.

Lemon ᵀᴵ
Cilantro ᵀᴵ
Juniper Berry ᵀᴵ
Bergamot ᵀᴵ
Siberian Fir ᵀᴵ

Gas (Flatulence)

Massage 1-3 drops into stomach area; take 1-3 drops internally as needed.

Fennel ᵀᴵ
Dill ᵀᴵ
Digestive Blend ᵀᴵ
Ginger ᵀᴵ
Tangerine ᵀᴵ

Protocol on pg. 163

Gastritis

Massage 1-3 drops into stomach area; take 1-2 drops internally diluted in carrier oil inside a veggie cap as needed.

Lavender ᵀᴵ
Ginger ᵀᴵ
Helichrysum ᵀᴵ
Jasmine ᵀ
Coriander ᵀᴵ

Protocol on pg. 163

Genital Warts

Dilute heavily with a carrier oil and apply 1-3 drops to affected area; take 1-3 drops internally a couple times daily.

Arborvitae ᵀ
Melissa ᵀᴵ
Frankincense ᵀᴵ
Thyme ᵀᴵ
Oregano ᵀᴵ

Giardia

Massage 1-3 drops clockwise onto stomach and chest area; take 1-3 drops internally as needed.

Oregano ᵀ ᴵ
Rosemary ᵀ ᴵ
Digestive Blend ᵀ ᴵ
Spearmint ᵀ ᴵ
Melaleuca ᵀ ᴵ

Gingivitis

Gargle 1-3 drops mixed with water several times daily; take 1-3 drops internally as needed.

Protective Blend ᵀ ᴵ
Clove ᵀ ᴵ
Melaleuca ᵀ ᴵ
Myrrh ᵀ ᴵ
Arborvitae ᵀ

Gluten Sensitivity

Take 1-3 drops internally as needed. Ingest Digestive Enzymes 20-30 minutes before eating, or during consumption.

Digestive Enzymes ᴵ
Digestive Blend ᵀ ᴵ
Lemongrass ᵀ ᴵ
Cardamom ᵀ ᴵ
Detoxification Blend ᵀ ᴵ

Gout

Take 1-3 drops internally twice a day; massage gently into affected joints as needed.

Lemongrass ᴬ ᵀ ᴵ
Wintergreen ᴬ ᵀ
Douglas Fir ᴬ ᵀ
Lemon ᴬ ᵀ ᴵ
Soothing Blend ᴬ ᵀ
Protocol on pg. 155

Growing Pains

Massage 1-3 drops into affected area as needed.

Lemongrass ᴬ ᵀ ᴵ
Marjoram ᴬ ᵀ ᴵ
Soothing Blend ᴬ ᵀ
Wintergreen ᴬ ᵀ
Spikenard ᴬ ᵀ ᴵ

Gum Disease

Apply 1-3 drops to gums; gargle a few drops in water as needed.

Clove ᵀ ᴵ
Myrrh ᵀ ᴵ
Protective Blend ᵀ ᴵ
Melaleuca ᵀ ᴵ
Geranium ᵀ ᴵ

Gums (Bleeding)

Apply 1-3 drops to gums; gargle with water as needed.

Myrrh ᵀ ᴵ
Helichrysum ᵀ ᴵ
Clove ᵀ ᴵ
Melaleuca ᵀ ᴵ
Geranium ᵀ ᴵ

Hair Loss

Dilute 5 drops in 20 drops of carrier oil. Massage a bit into scalp every night.

Rosemary ᵀ
Arborvitae ᵀ
Spikenard ᵀ
Cellular Complex ᵀ
Vitality Trio ᴵ

Halitosis

Gargle a few drops mixed with water several times daily or as needed; take 1-3 drops internally Cilantro twice daily.

Cilantro [I]
Protective Blend [I]
Spearmint [I]
Detoxification Blend [I]
Melaleuca [I]

Hand, Foot, & Mouth Disease

Apply 1-3 drops to affected areas (dilute for increased effectiveness).

Clove [A T]
Cellular Complex [A T]
Protective Blend [A T]
Melaleuca [A T]
Melissa [A T]

Hangover

Add 4-6 drops to warm bath; massage into back of neck and over liver; take 2-4 drops internally as needed.

Tension Blend [A T]
Digestive Blend [A T I]
Tangerine [A T I]
Detoxification Blend [A T I]
Encouraging Blend [A T]

Hay Fever

Apply 1-3 drops to back of neck, under nose, or chest as needed; take 1-3 drops internally of Cilantro, Petitgrain and Lemon; inhale from cupped hands.

Respiratory Blend [A T]
Cilantro [A T I]
Lemon [A T I]
Cleansing Blend [A T]
Petitgrain [A T I]
Protocol on pg. 154

Head Lice

Dilute 1-3 drops and apply to entire scalp, shampoo, and rinse 30 minutes later. Repeat daily for several days.

Melaleuca [T]
Arborvitae [T]
Outdoor Blend [T]
Rosemary [T]
Cleansing Blend [T]

Headache

Massage 1-3 drops into forehead, temples, and back of neck; inhale from cupped hands.

Tension Blend [A T]
Lavender [A T I]
Frankincense [A T I]
Rosemary [A T I]
Spearmint [A T I]

Hearing Issues

Apply 1-3 drops to temples and around the opening of the ear; apply to a cotton ball and place over ear opening overnight. Do NOT apply into ear.

Frankincense [T]
Helichrysum [T]
Melaleuca [T]
Basil [T]
Patchouli [T]

Heart Disease

Apply 1-3 drops over chest; take 1-3 drops internally as a daily supplement.

Marjoram [T I]
Geranium [T I]
Lemongrass [T I]
Helichrysum [T I]
Vitality Trio [I]

Heartburn

Massage 1-3 drops into abdomen; take 1-3 drops internally as needed.

Metabolic Blend [TI]
Digestive Blend [TI]
Ginger [TI]
Peppermint [TI]
Lavender [TI]
Protocol on pg. 164

Heat Exhaustion

Apply 1-3 drops to forehead, back of neck, inside of wrists, and bottom of feet; add Lemon or Peppermint to mineral water and sip slowly.

Tension Blend [AT]
Peppermint [ATI]
Lavender [ATI]
Siberian Fir [ATI]
Lemon [ATI]

Heatstroke

Apply 1-3 drops to forehead, temples, back of neck, and chest; take 1-3 drops internally as needed.

Peppermint [ATI]
Detoxification Blend [ATI]
Dill [ATI]
Tension Blend [AT]
Spearmint [ATI]

Heavy Metal Detox

Take 2-4 drops internally two times daily; massage 2-4 drops into bottoms of feet.

Cilantro [TI]
Frankincense [TI]
Cellular Complex [TI]
Detox Herbal Complex [I]
Black Pepper [TI]

Hematoma

Apply 1-3 to affected areas 2 to 3 times daily or as needed.

Cypress [T]
Massage Blend [T]
Geranium [T]
Marjoram [T]
Helichrysum [T]

Hemorrhoids

Dilute 2-4 drops with carrier oil and apply directly to affected areas daily or as needed.

Helichrysum [TI]
Myrrh [TI]
Cypress [T]
Geranium [TI]
Siberian Fir [TI]

Hepatitis

Take 1-3 drops internally; use topically with a warm compress over the liver area.

Geranium [ATI]
Myrrh [ATI]
Detoxification Blend [ATI]
Helichrysum [ATI]
Lavender [ATI]

Hernia (hiatal)

Massage 1-3 drops into affected area as needed.

Arborvitae [TI]
Helichrysum [TI]
Cypress [T]
Basil [TI]
Petitgrain [TI]

Herniated Disc

A T I

Massage 1-3 drops into affected area as needed.

Birch[T]
Lemongrass[TI]
Wintergreen[T]
Soothing Blend[T]
Polyphenol Complex[I]

Herpes Simplex

A T I

Take 1-3 drops internally; use topically with a warm compress over the kidney area; apply on the right and left side of throat daily.

Melissa[TI]
Protective Blend[TI]
Clove[TI]
Melaleuca[TI]
Oregano[TI]

Hiccups

A T I

Inhale 1-3 drops from cupped hands; massage into chest and stomach area as needed.

Arborvitae[AT]
Lemon[ATI]
Restful Bend[AT]
Digestive Blend[ATI]
Neroli[ATI]

HIV

A T I

Apply 1-3 drops to bottoms of feet; take 1-3 drops internally twice daily; inhale from cupped hands for emotional support.

Melissa[ATI]
Oregano[ATI]
Frankincense[ATI]
Melaleuca[ATI]
Myrrh[ATI]
Protocol on pg. 153

Hives

A T I

Apply 1-3 drops to affected area; take 2-4 drops internally twice daily as needed.

Melaleuca[TI]
Frankincense[TI]
Lavender[TI]
Peppermint[TI]
Spikenard[TI]

Hoarse Voice

A T I

Gargle 1-3 drops in water as needed; rub onto throat.

Lemon[ATI]
Myrrh[ATI]
Protective Blend[ATI]
Lavender[ATI]
Sandalwood[ATI]

Hormone Balance

A T I

Massage 1-3 drops into abdomen, temples, and bottoms of feet; ingest as needed; inhale from cupped hands.

Clary Sage[ATI]
Frankincense[ATI]
Ylang Ylang[ATI]
Sandalwood[ATI]
Juniper Berry[ATI]

Hot Flashes

A T I

Massage 1-3 drops into chest, neck, and face as needed; ingest Clary Sage and Ylang Ylang as needed.

Women's Blend[AT]
Women's Monthly[AT]
Clary Sage[ATI]
Ylang Ylang[ATI]
Jasmine[AT]
Protocol on pg. 167

Hyperactivity

Apply 1-3 drops on back of neck and bottoms of feet; inhale from cupped hands.

Cedarwood ^{A T}
Focus Blend ^{A T}
Vetiver ^{A T I}
Grounding Blend ^{A T}
Restful Blend ^{A T}

Hypertension

Apply 1-2 drops behind ears; inhale from cupped hands.

Grounding Blend ^{A T}
Wild Orange ^{A T I}
Yarrow ^{A T I}
Petitgrain ^{A T I}
Manuka ^{A T I}
Protocol on pg. 171

Hyperthyroid

Apply 1-3 drops to front of neck. Dilute with carrier oil for easier application. Take 1-3 drops internally a few times daily or as needed.

Frankincense ^{T I}
Rosemary ^{T I}
Myrrh ^{T I}
Detoxification Blend ^{T I}
Cellular Complex ^{T I}
Protocol on pg. 172

Hypoglycemia

Apply 1-3 drops to chest, bottoms of feet, and inside of wrists; take 1-3 drops internally a few times daily or as needed.

Metabolic Blend ^{T I}
Cinnamon ^{T I}
Coriander ^{T I}
Detoxification Blend ^{T I}
Cellular Complex ^{T I}

Hypothyroid

Apply 1-3 drops to front of neck. Dilute with carrier oil for easier application. Take 1-3 drops internally a few times daily or as needed.

Clove ^{T I}
Frankincense ^{T I}
Ginger ^{T I}
Lemongrass ^{T I}
Peppermint ^{T I}
Protocol on pg. 173

Immune Boost

Apply 2-4 drops to bottoms of feet; ingest as needed; inhale from cupped hands as needed.

Protective Blend ^{A T I}
Clove ^{A T I}
Melaleuca ^{A T I}
Oregano ^{A T I}
Black Pepper ^{A T I}
Protocol on pg. 165

Indigestion

Massage 1-3 drops into stomach area clockwise as needed.

Digestive Blend ^{T I}
Black Pepper ^{T I}
Metabolic Blend ^{T I}
Ginger ^{T I}
Wild Orange ^{T I}
Protocol on pg. 163

Infant Reflux

Dilute with carrier oil and apply 1-3 drops to stomach area and chest as needed.

Fennel ^T
Digestive Blend ^T
Dill ^T
Ginger ^T
Lavender ^T

Ailments

Infected Wounds

Apply 1-3 drops to affected areas 2 to 3 times daily as needed.

Myrrh ᵀ ᴵ
Helichrysum ᵀ ᴵ
Frankincense ᵀ ᴵ
Melaleuca ᵀ ᴵ
Cleansing Blend ᵀ ᴵ

Infertility

Apply 1-3 drops to abdomen daily; take 1-3 drops internally as needed.

Clary Sage ᴬ ᵀ ᴵ
Cellular Complex ᴬ ᵀ ᴵ
Ylang Ylang ᴬ ᵀ ᴵ
Detoxification Blend ᴬ ᵀ ᴵ
Vitality Trio ᴵ
Protocol on pg. 165

Inflammation

Apply 1-3 drops to affected areas as needed. For systemic inflammation, take 2-4 drops internally twice daily.

Wintergreen ᴬ ᵀ
Birch ᴬ ᵀ
Soothing Blend ᴬ ᵀ
Copaiba ᴬ ᵀ ᴵ
Spikenard ᴬ ᵀ ᴵ

Inflammatory Bowel Disease

Massage 1-3 drops into stomach; take internally as needed.

Spearmint ᴬ ᵀ ᴵ
Digestive Blend ᴬ ᵀ ᴵ
Detoxification Blend ᴬ ᵀ ᴵ
Ginger ᴬ ᵀ ᴵ
Lavender ᴬ ᵀ ᴵ
Protocol on pg. 165

Ingrown Toenail

Apply 1-3 drops to affected toenail as needed.

Ylang Ylang ᵀ
Cellular Complex ᵀ
Detoxification Blend ᵀ
Melaleuca ᵀ
Clove ᵀ

Insect Bites

Apply a drop or two to insect bite hourly or as needed.

Lavender ᵀ
Cleansing Blend ᵀ
Roman Chamomile ᵀ
Melaleuca ᵀ
Sandalwood ᵀ

Insomnia

Apply 1-3 drops to forehead, temples, base of skull, and behind the ear; diffuse.

Vetiver ᴬ ᵀ ᴵ
Restful Blend ᴬ ᵀ
Cedarwood ᴬ ᵀ
Petitgrain ᴬ ᵀ ᴵ
Restful Complex ᴵ
Protocol on pg. 170

Insulin Imbalance

Apply 1-3 drops to bottoms of feet and over pancreas; take a few drops internally as needed.

Oregano ᵀ ᴵ
Metabolic Blend ᵀ ᴵ
Coriander ᵀ ᴵ
Cleansing Blend ᵀ
Vitality Trio ᴵ
Protocol on pg. 162

Ailments

Irritable Bowels

Apply 1-3 drops to stomach as needed; take internally.

Digestive Blend [A][T][I]
Ginger [A][T][I]
Peppermint [A][T][I]
Spikenard [A][T][I]
Vetiver [A][T][I]
Protocol on pg. 165

Itchy Skin

Apply 1-3 drops to affected areas as needed. Use with carrier oil or lotion for improved efficacy.

Melaleuca [T][I]
Skin Clearing Blend [T]
Cedarwood [T]
Detoxification Blend [T][I]
Metabolic Blend [T][I]
Protocol on pg. 163

Jaundice

Massage 1-3 drops over the liver; take 1-3 drops internally as needed.

Detoxification Blend [A][T]
Geranium [A][T]
Rosemary [A][T]
Juniper Berry [A][T]
Cilantro [A][T]

Jet Lag

Apply 1-3 drops to forehead, temples, back of neck, and chest; inhale from cupped hands as needed.

Peppermint [A][T][I]
Tangerine [A][T][I]
Reassuring Blend [A][T]
Encouraging Blend [A][T]
Cellular Complex [A][T][I]

Jock Itch

Apply 1-3 drops to affected areas as needed with carrier oil; ingest a few drops as needed.

Melaleuca [T][I]
Thyme [T][I]
Patchouli [T][I]
Cleansing Blend [T]
Oregano [T][I]

Joint Pain

Massage 1-3 drops into affected areas as needed.

Wintergreen [A][T]
Soothing Blend [A][T]
Lemongrass [A][T][I]
Siberian Fir [A][T][I]
Polyphenol Complex [I]
Protocol on pg. 155

Kidney Infection

Apply 1-3 drops to kidney area a couple times daily; take 1-3 drops internally as needed.

Lemongrass [T][I]
Cinnamon [T][I]
Juniper Berry [T][I]
Protective Blend [T][I]
Cypress [T]

Kidney Stones

Massage 1-3 drops over kidney area; take 1-3 drops internally as needed.

Lemon [T][I]
Lemongrass [T][I]
Sandalwood [T][I]
Clary Sage [T][I]
Wintergreen [T]

Lactose Intolerance

Take 2-4 drops internally or massage into stomach as needed.

Digestive Blend ^{T I}
Coriander ^{T I}
Lemongrass ^{T I}
Digestive Enzymes ^I
Detoxification Blend ^{T I}

Laryngitis

Diffuse into the air and inhale 3 to 4 times daily or ingest a few drops as needed. Massage 1-3 drops on outside of throat.

Protective Blend ^{A T I}
Myrrh ^{A T I}
Lavender ^{A T I}
Frankincense ^{A T I}
Neroli ^{A T I}

Leg Cramps

Massage several drops into legs as needed.

Lemongrass ^{T I}
Cypress ^T
Soothing Blend ^T
Wintergreen ^T
Spikenard ^{T I}

Leukemia

Take 2-4 drops internally three times daily; massage into bottoms of feet as needed.

Frankincense ^{A T I}
Cellular Complex ^{A T I}
Lemongrass ^{A T I}
Detoxification Blend ^{A T I}
Geranium ^{A T I}

Libido (low)

Massage 1-3 drops into abdomen, bottoms of feet, and temples as needed; inhale from cupped hands as needed.

Ylang Ylang ^{A T I}
Women's Monthly ^{A T}
Inspiring Blend ^{A T}
Jasmine ^{A T}
Rose ^{A T}
Protocol on pg. 166

Lupus

Take 2-4 drops internally twice daily during flair ups; supplement regularly for long-term benefits.

Frankincense ^{A T I}
Cellular Complex ^{A T I}
Detoxification ^{A T I}
Polyphenol Complex ^I
Vitality Trio ^I
Protocol on pg. 166

Lyme Disease

Take 2-4 drops internally twice three times daily; supplement regularly for long-term benefits.

Cinnamon ^{A T I}
Oregano ^{A T I}
Clove ^{A T I}
Thyme ^{A T I}
Vitality Trio ^I
Protocol on pg. 166

Measles

Dab a few drops onto spots several times daily; add several drops to bath and soak for at least 30 minutes as needed.

Eucalyptus ^T
Melaleuca ^{T I}
Oregano ^{T I}
Lavender ^{T I}
Protective Blend ^{T I}

Melanoma

Apply 1-3 drops to affected areas; take 2-4 drops internally twice daily.

Arborvitae ᵀ ᴵ
Cedarwood ᵀ
Sandalwood ᵀ ᴵ
Cellular Complex ᵀ ᴵ
Clove ᵀ ᴵ

Memory Loss

Massage 1-3 drops into forehead, temples, back of neck, and chest as needed; inhale from cupped hands.

Rosemary ᴬ ᵀ ᴵ
Peppermint ᴬ ᵀ ᴵ
Focus Blend ᴬ ᵀ
Vetiver ᴬ ᵀ ᴵ
Frankincense ᴬ ᵀ ᴵ

Ailments

Meningitis

Take 2-4 drops internally twice daily; massage 2-4 drops into back of neck with carrier oil daily.

Melaleuca ᴬ ᵀ ᴵ
Lemongrass ᴬ ᵀ ᴵ
Protective Blend ᴬ ᵀ ᴵ
Basil ᴬ ᵀ ᴵ
Cellular Complex ᴬ ᵀ ᴵ

Menopause

Apply a few drops topically to abdomen, bottoms of feet, and back of neck daily; ingest Clary sage and Siberian fir as needed.

Clary Sage ᴬ ᵀ ᴵ
Women's Monthly ᴬ ᵀ
Siberian Fir ᴬ ᵀ ᴵ
Women's Blend ᴬ ᵀ
Cellular Complex ᴬ ᵀ ᴵ
Protocol on pg. 167

Menstrual Bleeding

Massage 2-4 drops into abdomen, lower back, and shoulders; apply to a warm compress over uterus area; take 2-4 drops internally as needed.

Helichrysum ᵀ ᴵ
Geranium ᵀ ᴵ
Clary Sage ᵀ ᴵ
Women's Monthly ᵀ
Detoxification Blend ᵀ ᴵ

Menstrual Pain

Massage 1-3 drops into abdomen, lower back, and shoulders; apply to a warm compress over uterus area; take 2-4 drops internally as needed.

Tension Blend ᴬ ᵀ
Clary Sage ᴬ ᵀ ᴵ
Women's Monthly ᴬ ᵀ
Marjoram ᴬ ᵀ ᴵ
Frankincense ᴬ ᵀ ᴵ
Protocol on pg. 167

Mental Fatigue

Massage 1-3 drops into forehead, temples, back of neck, and bottoms of feet; inhale from cupped hands as needed.

Peppermint ᴬ ᵀ ᴵ
Lemongrass ᴬ ᵀ ᴵ
Bergamot ᴬ ᵀ ᴵ
Invigorating Blend ᴬ ᵀ
Energy & Stamina ᴵ

Migraine

Apply 1-3 drops to forehead, temples, base of skull, back of neck, and bottoms of feet; inhale from cupped hands as needed.

Peppermint ᴬ ᵀ ᴵ
Marjoram ᴬ ᵀ ᴵ
Frankincense ᴬ ᵀ ᴵ
Tension Blend ᴬ ᵀ
Soothing Blend ᴬ ᵀ

Mold & Mildew

Diffuse into the air where mold is present several times daily until no longer needed. Mix 20 drops with 4 oz water and apply to area of concern.

Melaleuca ^{A T}
Cleansing Blend ^{A T}
Oregano ^{A T}
Arborvitae ^{A T}
Siberian Fir ^{A T}

Moles

Apply a drop to mole daily.

Oregano ^T
Frankincense ^T
Sandalwood ^T
Skin Clearing Blend ^T
Cellular Complex ^T

Mononucleosis

Take 1-3 drops internally twice a day; apply to bottoms of feet; diffuse.

Thyme ^{A T I}
Black Pepper ^{A T I}
Melissa ^{A T I}
Oregano ^{A T I}
Protective Blend ^{A T I}
Protocol on pg. 167

Mood Swings

Inhale 1-3 drops from cupped hands; apply a few drops to forehead, temples, back of neck, and bottoms of feet.

Patchouli ^{A T}
Restful Blend ^{A T}
Grounding Blend ^{A T}
Uplifting Blend ^{A T}
Renewing Blend ^{A T}

Morning Sickness

Apply 1-3 drops behind ears and over navel hourly; inhale from cupped hands; take 1-3 drops internally as needed.

Ginger ^{A T I}
Peppermint ^{A T I}
Digestive Blend ^{A T I}
Fennel ^{A T I}
Coriander ^{A T I}
Protocol on pg. 168

Motion Sickness

Apply 1-3 drops behind the ears and over navel; inhale from cupped hands; or take internally.

Ginger ^{A T I}
Grounding Blend ^{A T}
Peppermint ^{A T I}
Digestive Blend ^{A T I}
Basil ^{A T I}

Mouth Ulcers

Gargle 1-3 drops mixed with water several times daily; apply to gums; ingest as needed.

Protective Blend ^{T I}
Clove ^{T I}
Myrrh ^{T I}
Sandalwood ^{T I}
Melaleuca ^{T I}

Muscle Injury

Massage 1-3 drops into affected muscles as needed.

Marjoram ^{T I}
Basil ^{T I}
Soothing Blend ^T
Massage Blend ^T
Yarrow ^{T I}
Protocol on pg. 168

Muscle Pain

Massage 1-3 drops into affected muscles as needed.

Peppermint [T]
Soothing Blend [T]
Massage Blend [T]
Marjoram [T]
Soothing Blend [T]
Protocol on pg. 168

Muscle Spasms

Massage 1-3 drops into affected muscles as needed.

Basil [T]
Coriander [T]
Lemongrass [T]
Black Pepper [T]
Spikenard [T]

Muscle Stiffness

Massage 1-3 drops into affected muscles 2 to 3 times daily.

Massage Blend [T]
Tension Blend [T]
Lemongrass [T]
Siberian Fir [T]
Copaiba [T]
Protocol on pg. 168

Nasal Congestion

Apply 1-3 drops over bridge of nose, under nose, and rub over sinuses. Use carrier oil if desired.

Respiratory Blend [AT]
Siberian Fir [AT]
Digestion Blend [AT]
Eucalyptus [AT]
Peppermint [AT]

Nasal Polyps

Apply 1-3 drops over bridge of nose and under nose; take 1-3 drops internally twice daily.

Rosemary [ATI]
Melissa [ATI]
Respiratory Blend [AT]
Sandalwood [ATI]
Spikenard [ATI]

Nausea

Apply 1-3 drops behind ears and over navel hourly; place a drop under the tongue; inhale from cupped hands.

Ginger [ATI]
Digestion Blend [ATI]
Peppermint [ATI]
Detoxification Blend [ATI]
Grounding Blend [AT]

Neck Pain

Massage 1-3 drops onto neck several times daily. Blend with carrier oil to improve efficacy.

Soothing Blend [AT]
Birch [AT]
Wintergreen [AT]
Black Pepper [ATI]
Lemongrass [ATI]
Protocol on pg. 156

Nervous Fatigue

Inhale from cupped hands; apply 1-3 drops to temples, behind ears, and on back of neck as needed.

Arborvitae [AT]
Encouraging Blend [AT]
Cedarwood [AT]
Basil [AT]
Tangerine [AT]

37

Neuropathy

Apply 1-3 drops to affected areas several times daily; take 1-3 drops internally as needed.

Cypress [T]
Massage Blend [T]
Geranium [T I]
Soothing Blend [T]
Vetiver [T I]

Night Sweats

Apply 1-3 drops to abdomen and back of neck before sleeping.

Detox Herbal Complex [T]
Cellular Complex [T]
Lime [T]
Peppermint [T]
Tension Blend [T]

Nightmares

Apply 1-3 drops to abdomen and back of neck before sleeping; ingest as needed.

Juniper Berry [A T I]
Roman Chamomile [A T I]
Restful Blend [A T]
Petitgrain [A T I]
Comforting Blend [A T]

Nosebleeds

Apply 1-3 drops to the bridge and sides of nose and back of neck as needed.

Geranium [T I]
Helichrysum [T I]
Lavender [T I]
Myrrh [T I]
Soothing Blend [T]

Odors

Diffuse several drops; ingest 2-3 drops twice daily for body odors.

Cleansing Blend [A T]
Melaleuca [A T I]
Cilantro [A T I]
Arborvitae [A T]
Douglas Fir [A T]

Osteoarthritis

Apply 1-3 drops to affected areas daily.

Siberian Fir [T I]
Soothing Blend [T]
Wintergreen [T]
Lemongrass [T I]
Polyphenol Complex [I]

Osteoporosis

Massage 1-3 drops onto spine and affected areas daily; take Lemongrass internally.

Lemongrass [T I]
Clove [T I]
Wintergreen [T]
Cellular Complex [T I]
Bone Nutrient Complex [I]

Ovarian Cysts

Blend 1-3 drops with carrier oil and soak tampon, insert overnight; apply warm compress over the stomach; take internally.

Frankincense [T I]
Clary Sage [T I]
Basil [T I]
Sandalwood [T I]
Cellular Complex [T I]

38

Overeating

Apply 1-3 drops to stomach; take internally; inhale from cupped hands as needed.

Metabolic Blend ^{A T I} — Metabolic Blend ᴬᵀᴵ
Grapefruit ᴬᵀᴵ
Peppermint ᴬᵀᴵ
Renewing Blend ᴬᵀ
Cinnamon ᴬᵀᴵ

Protocol on pg. 173

Palpitations

Apply 1-3 drops to chest area as needed; inhale from cupped hands.

Geranium ᴬᵀᴵ
Wild Orange ᴬᵀᴵ
Ylang Ylang ᴬᵀᴵ
Marjoram ᴬᵀᴵ
Restful Blend ᴬᵀ

Pancreatitis

Take 1-3 drops internally several times weekly; massage 1-3 drops on abdomen as needed.

Detoxification Blend ᵀᴵ
Marjoram ᵀᴵ
Lemon ᵀᴵ
Coriander ᵀᴵ
Rosemary ᵀᴵ

Parasites

Take 2-4 drops internally; apply in a warm compress over intestinal area 2 to 3 times daily.

Detoxification Blend ᵀᴵ
Oregano ᵀᴵ
Digestive Blend ᵀᴵ
Clove ᵀᴵ
Thyme ᵀᴵ

Protocol on pg. 162

Pink Eye
(Conjunctivitis)

Apply a drop or two around (but not in) eyes. Rub in with carrier oil, being cautious around the eyes.

Melaleuca ᵀ
Rosemary ᵀ
Arborvitae ᵀ
Clary Sage ᵀ
Cleansing Blend ᵀ

Plantar Warts

Apply 1-3 drops to wart several times daily.

Cellular Complex ᵀ
Cleansing Blend ᵀ
Oregano ᵀ
Melissa ᵀ
Frankincense ᵀ

Pneumonia

Apply 1-3 drops to chest and neck area 3 to 5 times daily and gargle hourly; inhale from cupped hands as needed.

Protective Blend ᴬᵀᴵ
Arborvitae ᴬᵀ
Respiratory Blend ᴬᵀ
Bergamot ᴬᵀᴵ
Roman Chamomile ᴬᵀᴵ

Protocol on pg. 157

Poison Ivy/Oak

Apply 1-3 drops to affected area with carrier oil a couple times daily or as needed.

Frankincense ᵀ
Lavender ᵀ
Geranium ᵀ
Patchouli ᵀ
Petitgrain ᵀ

Post Traumatic Stress Disorder

Apply 1-3 drops to forehead, temples, back of neck, chest, and bottoms of feet; inhale from cupped hands as needed.

Cedarwood ^{A T}
Reassuring Blend ^{A T}
Sandalwood ^{A T}
Comforting Blend ^{A T}
Renewing Blend ^{A T}

PMS

Add 1-3 drops to warm bath; apply to abdomen; inhale from cupped hands; ingest Clary Sage and Geranium as needed.

Women's Monthly ^{A T}
Clary Sage ^{A T I}
Women's Blend ^{A T}
Frankincense ^{A T I}
Geranium ^{A T I}
Protocol on pg. 167

Prostatitis

Use 5-10 drops in a suppository nightly for 7 days or more, or massage 2-4 drops diluted onto perineum daily.

Rosemary ^{T I}
Thyme ^{T I}
Frankincense ^{T I}
Myrrh ^{T I}
Clary Sage ^{T I}

Psoriasis

Apply 1-3 drops to affected area a couple times daily with carrier oil; take 1-3 drops internally daily.

Melaleuca ^{A T I}
Thyme ^{A T I}
Roman Chamomile ^{A T I}
Detoxification Blend ^{A T I}
Probiotic Complex ^I
Protocol on pg. 169

Rashes

Dilute 1-3 drops with a carrier oil and apply to affected area as needed.

Arborvitae ^T
Roman Chamomile ^{T I}
Melaleuca ^{T I}
Cedarwood ^T
Lavender ^{T I}
Protocol on pg. 163

Respiratory Issues

Apply 1-3 drops to chest, neck, under nose, and on bridge of nose; inhale from cupped hands as needed.

Respiratory Blend ^{A T}
Eucalyptus ^{A T}
Douglas Fir ^{A T}
Cardamom ^{A T I}
Renewing Blend ^{A T}

Restless Leg Syndrome

Massage 1-3 drops onto legs before sleeping; inhale from cupped hands as needed.

Massage Blend ^{A T}
Wintergreen ^{A T}
Cypress ^{A T}
Petitgrain ^{A T}
Soothing Blend ^{A T}

Restlessness

Inhale from cupped hands; apply 1-3 drops to bottoms of feet and back of neck as needed.

Grounding Blend ^{A T}
Lavender ^{A T I}
Restful Blend ^{A T}
Vetiver ^{A T I}
Spikenard ^{A T I}

Rheumatic Fever

Apply 1-3 drops to bottoms of feet; take 1-3 drops internally twice daily; gargle a few drops mixed with water as needed.

Arborvitae [T]
Melissa [TI]
Wintergreen [T]
Oregano [TI]
Peppermint [TI]

Rhinitis

Inhale 1-3 drops from cupped hands several times daily; apply a couple drops to forehead and bridge of nose; take 1-2 drops internally.

Respiratory Blend [AT]
Melaleuca [ATI]
Peppermint [ATI]
Siberian Fir [ATI]
Oregano [ATI]

Ailments

Ringworm

Apply 1-3 drops to affected area 3-4 times daily.

Melaleuca [TI]
Cleansing Blend [T]
Skin Clearing Blend [T]
Petitgrain [TI]
Cedarwood [T]

Scarring

Massage a drop or two into scarred area 2 times daily.

Anti-Aging Blend [T]
Sandalwood [T]
Helichrysum [T]
Frankincense [T]
Yarrow [T]

Sciatica

Massage 1-3 drops into affected area a couple times daily.

Helichrysum [ATI]
Basil [ATI]
Vetiver [ATI]
Soothing Blend [AT]
Geranium [ATI]
Protocol on pg. 156

Seizures

Apply 1-3 drops to back of neck and bottoms of feet; inhale from cupped hands as needed; take 1-3 drops internally twice daily.

Spikenard [ATI]
Grounding Blend [AT]
Sandalwood [ATI]
Roman Chamomile [ATI]
Petitgrain [ATI]

Shingles

Apply 1-3 drops to affected area, on back of neck, and along the spine as needed; take 2-4 drops twice daily.

Black Pepper [TI]
Melissa [TI]
Melaleuca [TI]
Yarrow [TI]
Geranium [TI]
Protocol on pg. 169

Shock

Apply 1-3 drops on temples, under nose, and on back of neck as needed; inhale from cupped hands.

Grounding Blend [AT]
Helichrysum [AT]
Uplifting Blend [AT]
Renewing Blend [AT]
Tangerine [AT]

41

Ailments

Sinus Infection

Inhale 1-3 drops from cupped hands as needed; ingest a few drops; apply to chest, bridge of nose, and over sinuses with carrier oil.

Cardamom [A T I]
Respiratory Blend [A T]
Rosemary [A T I]
Siberian Fir [A T I]
Melissa [A T I]
Protocol on pg. 169

Smoking Addiction

Take 2-4 drops internally daily; inhale from cupped hands as needed when experiencing cravings.

Black Pepper [A T I]
Grapefruit [A T I]
Basil [A T I]
Bergamot [A T I]
Detoxification Blend [A T I]
Protocol on pg. 170

Sore Throat

Gargle 1-3 drops with water, then swallow; apply to throat and neck, diluting with carrier oil as needed.

Oregano [T I]
Protective Blend [T I]
Lemon [T I]
Arborvitae [T]
Melissa [T I]
Protocol on pg. 171

Stomach Ache

Apply 1-3 drops to stomach area as needed; take 1-3 drops internally as needed.

Ginger [T I]
Digestion Blend [T I]
Peppermint [T I]
Wild Orange [T I]
Roman Chamomile [T I]
Protocol on pg. 163

Skin Ulcers

Massage 1-3 drops into affected area a couple times daily. Dilute if necessary.

Arborvitae [T]
Myrrh [T]
Skin Clearing Blend [T]
Sandalwood [T]
Geranium [T]

Snoring

Apply 1-3 drops to chest and under nose; use in a diffuser beside bed at night.

Respiratory Blend [A T]
Petitgrain [A T]
Vetiver [A T]
Eucalyptus [A T]
Douglas Fir [A T]
Protocol on pg. 171

Sprains

Gently apply 1-3 drops to affected area as needed.

Soothing Blend [T]
Helichrysum [T]
Lemongrass [T]
Spikenard [T]
Massage Blend [T]

Stretch Marks

Massage 1-3 drops into affected areas a couple times daily.

Anti-Aging Blend [T]
Sandalwood [T]
Myrrh [T]
Neroli [T]
Spikenard [T]

Stroke

Apply 1-3 drops on temples, forehead, behind ears, and back of neck; take 1-2 drops internally twice daily.

Fennel ^{A T I}
Cypress ^{A T}
Helichrysum ^{A T I}
Basil ^{A T I}
Cinnamon ^{A T I}

Sunburn

Apply 1-3 drops to affected area hourly or as needed. Blend 2-3 oils, 2-3 drops each with carrier oil, for improved results.

Lavender ^T
Helichrysum ^T
Peppermint ^T
Cedarwood ^T
Frankincense ^T
Protocol on pg. 172

Teething Pain

Dilute with carrier oil and gently massage a drop along baby's jawline, reapplying as needed.

Lavender ^T
Clove ^T
Wintergreen ^T
Frankincense ^T
Spikenard ^T

Tendinitis

Massage 1-3 drops onto affected areas 4 to 5 times daily, or as needed.

Lemongrass ^{T I}
Cardamom ^{T I}
Marjoram ^{T I}
Soothing Blend ^T
Polyphenol Complex ^I

Tennis Elbow

Massage 1-3 drops onto affected area as needed.

Lemongrass ^{T I}
Soothing Blend ^{T I}
Siberian Fir ^{T I}
Blue Tansy ^{T I}
Frankincense ^{T I}

Testosterone (low)

Apply 2-4 drops to bottoms of feet twice daily; inhale from cupped hands as needed.

Patchouli ^{A T I}
Sandalwood ^{A T I}
Inspiring Blend ^{A T}
Focus Blend ^{A T}
Rose ^{A T}

Thrush

Gargle 1-3 drops mixed with water several times daily; apply topically to lower throat and bottoms of feet; take 1-3 drops internally as needed.

Lemon ^{T I}
Wild Orange ^{T I}
Arborvitae ^T
Oregano ^{T I}
Protective Blend ^{T I}
Protocol on pg. 172

Tick Bites

Apply 1-2 drops to bite frequently for the first hour after carefully removing tick. Dilute Oregano if necessary.

Melaleuca ^T
Outdoor Blend ^T
Cleansing Blend ^T
Lavender ^T
Oregano ^T

Ailments

Tinnitus

Apply 1-2 drops behind ear 2-3 times daily.

Grounding Blend [T]
Helichrysum [T]
Basil [T]
Rosemary [T]
Cypress [T]

Tonsillitis

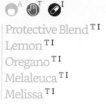

Gargle 1-3 drops mixed with water or ingest; apply to throat and chest several times daily. Dilute if necessary.

Protective Blend [T I]
Lemon [T I]
Oregano [T I]
Melaleuca [T I]
Melissa [T I]

Toothache

Apply a drop to gums or ingest by adding to water, gargling, and swallowing daily, or as needed.

Clove [T I]
Melaleuca [T I]
Protective Blend [T I]
Helichrysum [T I]
Wintergreen [T]

Trauma (Emotional)

Apply 2-4 drops to forehead, temples, back of neck, and chest; inhale from cupped hands as needed.

Renewing Blend [A T]
Reassuring Blend [A T]
Grounding Blend [A T]
Comforting Blend [A T]
Rose [A T]

Ulcers (Stomach)

Take 1-3 drops internally at least once daily; massage gently into abdomen as needed.

Detoxification Blend [T I]
Lemongrass [T I]
Myrrh [T I]
Frankincense [T I]
Geranium [T I]

Urinary Tract Infection

Massage 1-3 drops over the kidneys and on bottoms of the feet; take interally as needed.

Cypress [T]
Basil [T I]
Cleansing Blend [T]
Lemongrass [T I]
Juniper Berry [T I]

Varicose Veins

Massage 1-3 drops into the affected area several times daily.

Helichrysum [T]
Cardamom [T]
Cypress [T]
Siberian Fir [T]
Detoxification Blend [T]

Vision Loss

Apply 1-3 drops around the opening of the eye or apply to a cotton ball and place over eye. Do NOT apply into eye.

Anti-Aging Blend [T]
Clary Sage [T]
Cellular Complex [T]
Helichrysum [T]
Focus Blend [T]

Ailments

Vomiting

Apply 1-3 drops to stomach area as needed; inhale from cupped hands.

Digestive Blend ATI
Peppermint ATI
Ginger ATI
Bergamot ATI
Roman Chamomile ATI

Warts (common)

Apply a drop directly to wart several times daily until the wart disappears. Avoid the surrounding skin with Oregano.

Oregano T
Thyme T
Frankincense T
Skin Clearing Blend T
Neroli T

Wasp Sting

Apply one drop to sting several times daily or as needed.

Lavender T
Cleansing Blend T
Roman Chamomile T
Myrrh T
Cedarwood T

Weight Loss

Add 1-3 drops to water to manage cravings and encourage metabolism. Inhale from cupped hands to satisfy cravings.

Metabolic Blend ATI
Grapefruit ATI
Peppermint ATI
Lemon ATI
Energy & Stamina I
Protocol on pg. 173

Whiplash

Massage 1-3 drops into affected area as needed. Use with carrier oil to improve efficacy.

Soothing Blend T
Siberian Fir T
Lemongrass T
Patchouli T
Sandalwood T

Withdrawal Symptoms

Apply 1-3 drops to bottoms of feet and back of neck; inhale from cupped hands as needed; add 1-3 drops to water.

Cilantro ATI
Cinnamon ATI
Juniper Berry ATI
Detoxification Blend ATI
Encouraging Blend AT

Worms

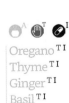

Apply 2-4 drops to stomach area and on bottoms of feet 2 or 3 times daily; ingest 2-3 drops twice daily.

Oregano TI
Thyme TI
Ginger TI
Basil TI
Clove TI

Wrinkles

Apply 1-3 drops to the affected areas as needed. Add to facial lotion or use with carrier oil for added benefits.

Anti-Aging Blend T
Geranium T
Frankincense T
Spikenard T
Cedarwood T

Section 3

Emotional
Uses

Emotional Uses

The chemical constituents in oils can trigger a quick change in brain chemistry, and a fast improvement in emotions. This emotional use guide groups three related emotions, and pairs them with three oils to promote a healthier emotional state.

Use one or more of the suggested oils with these methods of application. Find what feels best for you.

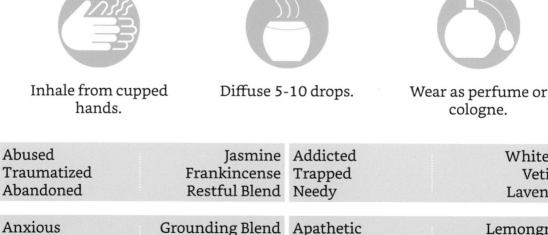

Inhale from cupped hands.

Diffuse 5-10 drops.

Wear as perfume or cologne.

Abused	Jasmine	Addicted	White Fir
Traumatized	Frankincense	Trapped	Vetiver
Abandoned	Restful Blend	Needy	Lavender
Anxious	Grounding Blend	Apathetic	Lemongrass
Panicking	Tension Blend	Disinterested	Detoxification Blend
Flustered	Neroli	Bored	Lime
Bitter	Cardamom	Confused	Roman Chamomile
Angry	Thyme	Distracted	Focus Blend
Resentful	Siberian Fir	Purposeless	Peppermint

Controlled	Blue Tansy	Depressed	Joyful Blend
Powerless	Clove	Discouraged	Hopeful Blend
Shameful	Grapefruit	Disheartened	Melissa
Distressed	Tangerine	Gloomy	Uplifting Blend
Worried	Reassuring Blend	Sad	Invigorating Blend
Fearful	Black Pepper	Somber	Respiratory Blend
Grieving	Helichrysum	Insecure	Inspiring Blend
Wounded	Ylang Ylang	Unconfident	Bergamot
Hurt	Comforting Blend	Self-conscious	Coriander
Materialistic	Cilantro	Pessimistic	Bergamot
Inauthentic	Fennel	Irritable	Women's Monthly
Irresponsible	Ginger	Self-loathing	Metabolic Blend
Prideful	Cinnamon	Stubborn	Wintergreen
Jealous	Oregano	Unyielding	Juniper Berry
Controlling	Sandalwood	Inflexible	Arborvitae
Uncertain	Copaiba	Unloving	Geranium
Self-deceiving	Patchouli	Withholding	Rose
Over Stimulated	Spearmint	Unforgiving	Renewing Blend
Unmotivated	Encouraging Blend	Unsupported	Birch
Discontented	Wind Orange	Lonely	Lemon
Lethargic	Cypress	Indecisive	Cedarwood

Section 4

Single
Oils

Arborvitae
Thuja Plicata

Application

 A   T   I

Chemical Constituents
a, B, y-thujaplicin
Methyl thujate
Thujic acid

Other Uses
Colds, Cold Sores, Cysts, Fevers, Intestinal Parasites, Meditation, Respiratory Viruses

Top *Uses*

1 Strep Throat
Rub 2 drops over outside of throat, and gargle 2 drops with water.

2 Bug Repellent
Dillute with several drops of carrier oil, and rub over needed areas.

3 Skin Cancer
Apply diluted to the affected area often and in small amounts.

4 Candida
Rub 2 drops over abdomen and bladder several times a day.

5 Fungal Issues
Apply neat to needed areas.

6 Furniture Polish
Combine 4 drops with 4 drops lemon oil, and rub in using a clean rag.

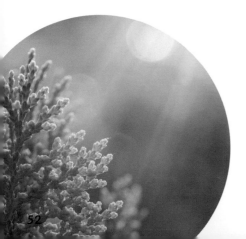

Basil
Ocimum Basilicum

Application

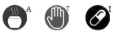

Chemical Constituents
Linalool
Methyl chavicol
1, 8 cineol

Other Uses
Bee Stings, Bronchitis, Dizziness, Frozen Shoulder, Gout, Greasy Hair, Infertility, Lactation (increase milk supply), Loss of Sense of Smell, Migraines, Nausea, Viral Hepatitis

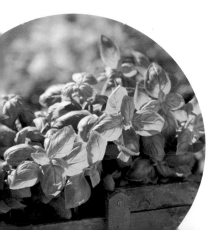

Top *Uses*

1 Adrenal Fatigue
Apply 1-2 drops directly to the adrenal areas or to the bottoms of the feet.

2 Mental Fatigue
Inhale from cupped hands, or diffuse.

3 Earache
Place a drop on a cotton ball, and rest over the ear for 15 minutes.

4 Muscle Spasms
Massage into muscles with carrier oil.

5 Carpal Tunnel
Massage into wrists & joints.

6 Cramps (abdominal)
Rub a drop clockwise over abdomen.

7 Cooking
Use a toothpick to add to dishes according to taste.

Bergamot
Citrus Bergamia

Application
 A 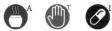 T I

Chemical Constituents
d-limonene
Lilayl acetate
Linalol

Other Uses
Brain Injury, Colic, Depression, Fungus
Issues, Irritability, Low Energy, Muscle
Cramps, Oily Skin, Stress

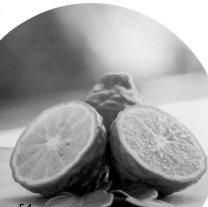

Safety
Avoid sun for
12 hours after
topical appli-
cation.

Top *Uses*

1 Psoriasis
*Dilute 1-2 drops heavily with carrier oil,
and apply frequently to affected area.*

2 Sadness
Inhale from cupped hands or diffuse.

3 Appetite Loss
*Drink 1-2 drops in 8 oz. water throughout
the day, or diffuse.*

4 Addictions
Apply to bottoms of feet, or diffuse.

5 Acne
*Apply small amount to affected areas.
Avoid sun for 12 hours after.*

6 Self-Confidence/Self-Worth
Apply over sacral (belly button).

7 Insomnia
Use 1 drop under tongue or in water.

Birch
Betula Lenta

Application

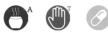

Chemical Constituents
Methyl salicylate
Betulene
Betulinol

Other Uses
Cramps, Gout, Joint Pain, Gallbladder Stones, Kidney Stones, Ulcers

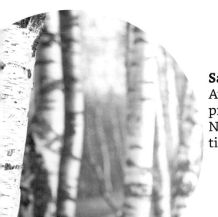

Safety
Avoid during pregnancy. Not for epileptics.

Top *Uses*

1 Broken bones
Massage 2 drops over and around affected area, avoiding open wounds.

2 Arthritis & Rheumatism
Massage 1-2 drops into affected area.

3 Muscle Aches
Massage 1-2 drops with carrier oil or lotion into muscles.

4 Whiplash
Gently massage with carrier oil. Consider using in Swedish massage.

5 Connective Tissue Injury
Apply neat to affected area.

6 Fever
Apply neat or diluted to back of neck.

7 Bone Spurs
Apply neat to areas of concern.

Single Oils

Black Pepper
Piper Nigrum

Application

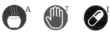

Chemical Constituents
l-limonene
B-caryophyllene
Caryophyllene oxide

Other Uses
Antioxidant, Anxiety, Cellular Oxygenation, Diarrhea, Digestion, Gas, Emotional Repression, Inflammation, Laxative

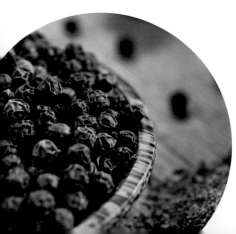

Safety
Dilute for use on sensitive skin.

Top *Uses*

1 Cold & Flu
Take 2 drops in a capsule, or apply to the bottoms of feet.

2 Smoking (quitting)
Apply to bottoms of feet (big toes) several times a day to curb cravings.

3 Circulation
Apply to bottoms of feet.

4 Sprains
Massage into muscles with carrier oil.

5 Congestion
Apply diluted over chest and upper back.

6 Airborne Viruses
Diffuse to cleanse the air.

7 Cooking
Add a drop to soups, sauces, and other dishes.

Blue Tansy
Tanacetum Annuum

Application
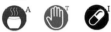

Chemical Constituents
Sabinene
Chamazulene
Camphor

Other Uses
Bacterial Infection, Constipation, Cramping, Eczema, Fungus, Gas, Gout, Indigestion, Insect Repellent, Psoriasis, Rashes, Rheumatism, Sneezing

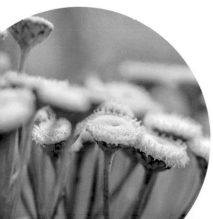

Safety
Dilute for use on sensitive skin.

Top *Uses*

1 Allergies
Put 1-2 drops under the tongue, then swallow with water after 30 seconds.

2 Arthritis & Muscle Pain
Add 5-10 drops to a bath, or massage into affected areas with carrier oil.

3 Anxiety
Apply a drop to pulse points, or diffuse.

4 Digestive Discomfort
Massage 2 drops clockwise onto stomach.

5 Dry, Itchy, or Inflamed Skin
Apply heavily diluted to affected skin.

6 Headaches
Rub a drop into temples and back of skull.

7 Congestion
Rub 2 drops onto chest and mid-back.

Cardamom
Elettaria Cardamomum

Application

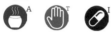

Chemical Constituents
a-terpenyl accetate
Linalol
Sabinene

Other Uses
Colitis, Constipation, Headaches, Inflammation, Menstrual Pain, Muscle Aches, Nausea, Pancreatitis, Respiratory Issues, Sore Throat, Stomach Ulcers

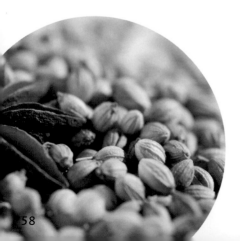

Top *Uses*

1 Digestive Discomfort
Drink a drop with a glass of water or in a capsule, or rub over stomach.

2 Congestion
Rub with carrier oil over chest, or diffuse.

3 Indigestion
Drink a drop with water or in a capsule.

4 Cough
Rub with carrier oil over chest.

5 Motion Sickness
Put a drop under the tongue.

6 Asthma, Shortness of Breath
Apply to bottoms of feet or over chest.

7 Cooking
Use a toothpick to add to dishes according to taste.

Cassia
Cinnamomum Cassia

Application
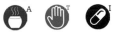

Chemical Constituents
Trans-cinnamaldehyde
Eugenol
Cinnamyl accetate

Other Uses
Antiseptic, Boils, Circulation, Cold Limbs,
Upset Stomach, Typhoid

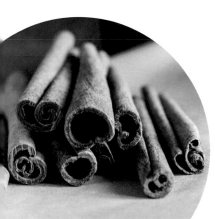

Safety
Dilute heavily
for topical use.
Avoid during
pregnancy.

Top *Uses*

1 Vomiting
*Take 1-2 drops in a capsule to restore
proper digestion.*

2 Viruses & Bacteria
*Diffuse to cleanse the air, or take 1-2
drops in a capsule to combat internally.*

3 Water Retention
*Apply to bottoms of feet, take 1-2 drops
in a capsule, or add 2 drops to bath.*

4 Blood Sugar Balance
Take 1-2 drops in capsule with food.

5 Sex Drive
Use heavily diluted in massage, or diffuse.

6 Metabolism Boost
Apply to adrenal reflex points.

7 Cooking
Use a toothpick to add to dishes.

Cedarwood
Juniperus Virginiana

Application

Chemical Constituents
A & B-Cedrene
Trans-caryophyllene
Cedrol

Other Uses
Blemishes, Cough, Dandruff, Gums, Insect Repellent, Respiratory Function, Sinusitis, Vaginal Infection, Tension

Safety
Cedarwood is very mild, and safe for even the most sensitive skin.

Top *Uses*

1 Eczema & Psoriasis
Apply neat and often to affected areas.

2 ADD/ADHD
Apply to wrists, temples, and back of neck, or diffuse.

3 Sleep
Rub onto bottoms of feet and back of neck, and diffuse. Blend with Lavender.

4 Anxiety
Apply to wrists and temples.

5 Cuts & Scrapes
Apply around wounded area to promote healing.

6 Urinary & Bladder Infection
Apply over bladder.

7 Seizers & Stroke
Apply to back of neck and bottoms of feet.

Cilantro
Coriandrum Sativum

Application

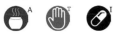

Chemical Constituents
Tetradecanal
Cyclododecanol
Eugenol

Other Uses
Allergies, Antioxidant, Anxiety, Bloating, Gas, Liver Support, Kidney Support

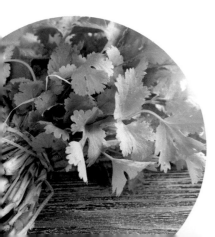

Top *Uses*

1 Heavy Metal Detox
Apply to the bottoms of feet morning and night.

2 Halitosis
Take 1-2 drops in capsule.

3 Detox
Apply over liver, kidneys, and bottoms of feet.

4 Fungal Infections
Take 1-2 drops in a capsule for internal issues, or apply topically for external issues.

5 Body Odor
Use small amounts in food, or take 1-2 drops in a capsule to deodorize internally.

6 Cooking
Use a toothpick to add to dishes according to taste.

Single Oils

61

Cinnamon
Cinnamomum Zeylanicum

Application

Chemical Constituents
Trans-cinnamaldeyde
Eugenol
Linalol

Other Uses
Airborne Bacteria, Cholesterol, Diverticulitis, Fungal Infections, General Tonic, Immune Support, Pancreas Support, Pneumonia, Typhoid, Vaginitis

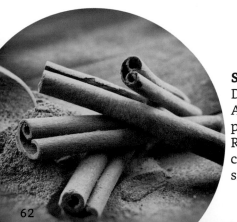

Safety
Dilute heavily. Avoid during pregnancy. Repeated use can cause sensitivity.

Top *Uses*

1 High Blood Sugar
Take 1-2 drops in capsule, or drink with large glass of water.

2 Bacterial Infection
Apply heavily diluted for external infection, or take 1-2 drops in capsule for internal infection.

3 Sex Drive
Use heavily diluted in massage, or diffuse.

4 Cavities
Swish a drop with water as a mouthwash.

5 Diabetes
Take 1-2 drop in a capsule daily.

6 Alkalinity
Drink in water to promote alkalinity.

7 Cooking
Use a toothpick to achieve desired flavor.

Clary Sage
Salvia Sclarea

Application
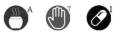

Chemical Constituents
Linalyl acetate
Linalol
Sclareol

Other Uses
Aneurysm, Breast Enlargement, Cholesterol, Convulsions, Endometriosis, Epilepsy, Fragile Hair, Hot Flashes, Impotence, Lactation, Parkinson's, Premenopause, Seizure

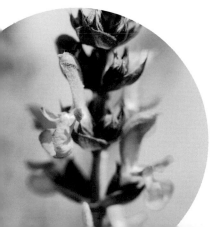

Safety
Use with caution during pregnancy.

Top *Uses*

1 Hormone Balance
Apply to wrists and behind ears.

2 PMS
Apply to bottoms of feet, or take 1-2 drops in capsule.

3 Postpartum Depression
Diffuse or apply over heart area.

4 Abdominal Cramps
Massage over abdomen.

5 Pink Eye
Apply carefully around edge of eye.

6 Infertility
Apply to abdomen & uterine reflex points, or take 1-2 drops in capsule.

7 Breast Cancer
Apply diluted to breasts, or take 1-2 drops in capsule to regulate estrogen levels.

Clove
Eugenia Caryophyllata

Application

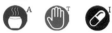 A   T   I

Chemical Constituents
Eugenol
Eugenyl Acetate
B-caryophyllene

Other Uses
Addictions, Blood Clots, Candida, Cataracts, Fever, Herpes Simplex, Hodgkin's Disease, Glaucoma, Gingivitis, Lipoma, Lupus, Lyme Disease, Macular Degeneration, Memory Loss, Parasites, Termites

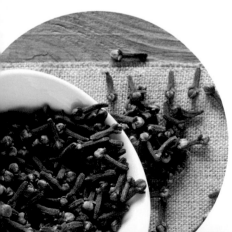

Safety
Can irritate sensitive skin. Use with caution during pregnancy.

Top *Uses*

1 Thyroid (hypo, Hashimoto's)
Apply diluted over thyroid or to thyroid reflex point, or take 1-2 drops in capsule.

2 Toothache
Apply directly to problematic tooth.

3 Smoking Addiction
Rub onto bottom of big toe.

4 Immune Support
Take 1-2 drops in a capsule.

5 Antioxidant
Take 1-2 drops in a capsule, or use in cooking.

6 Liver Detox
Rub over liver or on liver reflex point.

7 Rheumatoid Arthritis
Massage diluted into affected area.

Copaiba
Copaifera Officinalis

Application

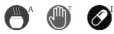

Chemical Constituents
d-Limonene
y-terpinene
Lilayl acetate

Other Uses
Anxiety, Congestion, Infection, Mood Disorders, Nail Fungus, Skin Strengthening

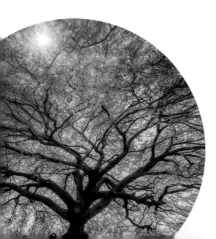

Top *Uses*

1 Headache & Migraine
Massage gently onto temples, scalp, and the back of the neck.

2 Pain & Inflammation
Inhale or diffuse, or apply topically to affected areas.

3 Wrinkles, Pimples, Blisters
Apply daily with a carrier oil.

4 High Blood Pressure
Apply to the bottoms of feet twice daily.

5 Athlete's Foot
Apply several drops to clean, dry feet.

6 Detox
Apply over bladder to stimulate detox through urination.

Coriander
Coriandrum Sativum

Application

 A T ⬤ I

Chemical Constituents
Linalol
a-pinene
Geranyl

Other Uses
Alzheimer's, Itchy Skin, Joint Pain, Low Energy, Measles, Muscle Tone, Muscle Spasms, Nausea, Neuropathy, Stiffness, Whiplash

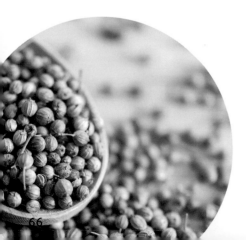

Top *Uses*

1 Diabetes (high blood sugar)
Combine with 1 drop Cinnamon & Juniper Berry in capsule daily.

2 Food Poisoning
Drink 2 drops in water, or take in capsule.

3 Body Odor
Drink 2 drops in water, or take in capsule.

4 Cartilage Injury
Massage into affected area with carrier oil.

5 Rashes
Apply diluted to affected area.

6 Muscle Aches
Take a drop in a capsule, or massage with carrier oil onto affected muscles.

7 Cooking
Use a toothpick to add desired flavor.

Single Oils

Cumin
Cuminum Cyminum

Application

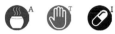

Chemical Constituents
Cuminaldehyde
Beta-pinene,
Para-cymene

Other Uses
Skin Warming

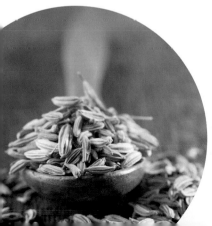

Safety
Possible skin
sensitivity.
Avoid sun for
12 hours after
topical appli-
cation.

Top *Uses*

1 Flatulence
Take 1-2 drops in capsule.

2 Cooking
Use a toothpick to add to dishes according to taste. Especially good for stews, soups, dressings, and sauces.

3 Digestive Discomfort
Take 1-2 drops in a capsule.

4 Organ Detox
Take 1-2 drops in a capsule daily for 3-5 days.

5 Mouth Rinse
Swish a drop with water as a natural mouthwash.

Cypress
Cupressus Sempervirens

Application

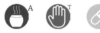

Chemical Constituents
a-pinene
Cedrol
a-terpinyl acetate

Other Uses
Aneurysm, Bunions, Edema, Hemorrhoids, Flu, Incontinence, Lou Gehrig's Disease, Ovary Issues, Prostate Issues, Raynaud's Disease, Tuberculosis, Varicose Veins, Whooping Cough

Safety
Can irritate sensitive skin. Use with caution during pregnancy.

Top *Uses*

1 Circulation (poor)
Apply 2 drops to the bottoms of each foot morning and night.

2 Bladder/Urinary Tract Infection
Massage 2 drops with carrier oil over bladder. Repeat every 2 hours as needed.

3 Bone Spurs
Apply directly onto affected area.

4 Concussion
Massage 2 drops with carrier oil into back of neck, back of skull, and shoulders.

5 Restless Leg Syndrome
Massage 2 drops with carrier oil into bottoms of feet, calves, and upper legs.

6 Bed Wetting
Apply 2 drops neat over bladder before bed.

Dill
Anethum Graveolens

Application

Chemical Constituents
d-limonene
d-arvone
a & b-phellandrene

Other Uses
Colic, Dyspepsia, Electrolyte Imbalance,
Flatulence, Indigestion, Insulin Imbalance,
Liver Deficiency, Nervousness, Pancreas
Support

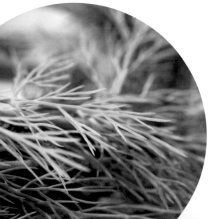

Safety
Use with
caution when
epileptic.

Top *Uses*

1 Cholesterol
*Apply to arches of feet, or take 1-2 drops
in a capsule.*

2 Flavoring
*Use a toothpick to achieve desired flavor
in dips and sauces.*

3 Constipation
Take 1-2 drops in a capsule.

4 Lactation (increase milk supply)
*Take 1-2 drops in a capsule, or massage
with carrier oil around breast.*

5 Missing Menstrual Cycle
Rub 1 drop with carrier oil over abdomen.

6 Muscle Spasms
*Massage with carrier oil over agitated or
overactive muscles.*

Douglas Fir
Pseudotsuga Menziesil

Application

Chemical Constituents
Linalol
a-pinene
Geranyl

Other Uses
Arthritis, Constipation, Depression, Emotional Congestion, Energy, Generational Patterns, Weight Gain, Sinus Issues

Top *Uses*

1 Muscle Soreness
Rub 2-4 drops with carrier oil onto sore muscles.

2 Congestion
Rub 1-2 drops over chest, or diffuse.

3 Headache & Migraine
Rub a drop into temples.

4 Focus & Mental Clarity
Inhale from cupped hands, or diffuse.

5 Skin Irritations
Apply heavily diluted to irritated skin.

6 Household Cleansing
Use with Lemon oil for a refreshing household cleaner.

7 Cough
Apply 1-2 drops to chest or lung reflex points.

Eucalyptus
Eucalyptus Radiata

Application

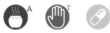

Chemical Constituents
1,8 ceneol
a & B-pinenes
a-terpineol

Other Uses
Colds, Fever, Flu, Headache, Earaches, Insect Bites & Stings, Kidney Stones, Muscle Aches, Neuralgia, Rheumatism, Rhinitis

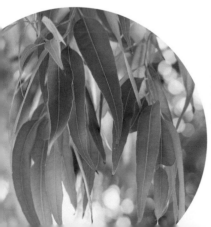

Safety
Not for use topically on newborns.

Top *Uses*

1 Congestion & Cough
Apply 2-4 drops to chest, or diffuse.

2 Bronchitis & Pneumonia
Apply 2-4 drops to chest & mid-back, or diffuse.

3 Sinusitis
Apply heavily diluted to sinuses, carefully avoiding eyes.

4 Asthma
Inhale 2 drops from cupped hands, and apply to lung reflex points.

5 Menstrual Cramp
Rub 1-2 drops with carrier oil over abdomen.

6 Mental Fatigue
Inhale 1-2 drops from cupped hands, or diffuse.

Fennel
Foeniculum Vulgare

Single Oils

Application
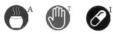

Chemical Constituents
Trans-anethole
Trans-ocimene
Linalol

Other Uses
Blood Sugar Imbalance, Constipation, Digestive Disorders, Edema, Fertility Issues, Fluid Retention, Intestinal Parasites, Menopause, PMS, Spasms, Stroke

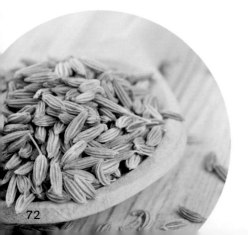

Top *Uses*

1 Flatulence
Rub 1-2 drops over outside of stomach, or drink with water.

2 Milk Supply (low)
Massage 1 drop diluted around nipples 2-3 times daily.

3 Digestive Disorders
Drink 1-2 drops in water or capsule.

4 Nausea
Rub 1-2 drops over stomach, or drink a drop in water.

5 Menstrual Discomfort
Rub a drop over abdomen.

6 Parasites
Drink 2-4 drops in a capsule.

7 Colic
Rub a drop diluted over stomach.

Frankincense
Boswellia Frereana

Application
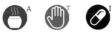

Chemical Constituents
a-phellandrenes
B-elemene
Cis-verbenol

Other Uses
ADHD, Aneurysm, Asthma, Balance, Brain Health, Coma, Concussion, Fibroids, Genital Warts, Immune Support, Lou Gehrig's Disease, Memory, Moles, MRSA, Multiple Sclerosis, Scarring, Sciatica, Warts, Wrinkles

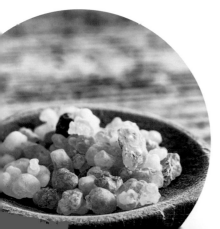

Top *Uses*

1 Depression & Anxiety
Use a drop under the tongue, apply to pulse points, or diffuse.

2 Alzheimer's & Dementia
Apply 2 drops to bottoms of feet and base of skull twice daily.

3 Cellular Function
Take 1-2 drops in capsule.

4 Pain & Inflammation
Use a drop under the tongue, or massage into inflamed areas.

5 Parkinson's
Apply 1-2 drops to brain reflex points, and diffuse.

6 Cancer
Take 1-2 drops in capsule, and apply close to the affected area frequently.

Geranium
Pelargonium Graveolens

Application

 A T I

Chemical Constituents
Citronellol
Citronellyl Formate
Isomenthone

Other Uses
Autism, Bleeding, Circulation, Depression, Diarrhea, Gastric Ulcers, Hernia, Low Libido, Menstrual Cramps, Menopause, Neuralgia, Raynaud's Disease, Spasms, Vertigo

Safety
Possible skin sensitivity.

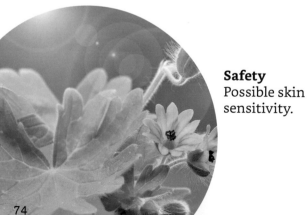

Top *Uses*

1 **Liver & Kidney Support**
Rub a drop directly over liver and kidneys.

2 **Autism**
Apply 1-2 drops to bottoms of feet, or diffuse.

3 **Jaundice**
Apply 1 drop diluted to bottoms of feet, and diffuse.

4 **PMS & Hormone Balance**
Apply a drop to pulse points.

5 **Hemorrhoids**
Apply heavily diluted to affected areas.

6 **Reproductive Disorders (female)**
Apply 1-2 drops to reproductive reflex points.

7 **Varicose Veins**
Massage diluted into affected areas.

Ginger
Zingiber Officinale

Application

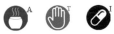

Chemical Constituents
Zingiberene
Camphene
Nonanol

Other Uses
Aneurysm, Breast Enlargement, Cholesterol, Convulsions, Endometriosis, Epilepsy, Fragile Hair, Hot Flashes, Impotence, Lactation, Parkinson's, Premenopause, Seizure

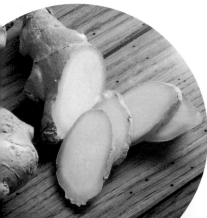

Safety
Possible skin sensitivity.

Top *Uses*

1 Nausea & Stomach Upset
Drink 1-2 drops in capsule.

2 Vomiting
Rub a drop heavily diluted over stomach.

3 Constipation
Apply 1-2 drops diluted over stomach, or take in capsule.

4 Immune Support
Apply 1-2 drops to bottoms of feet, or drink in capsule.

5 Congestion & Cough
Diffuse 3-6 drops.

6 Cold & Flu
Apply 1-2 drops to bottoms of feet, or drink in capsule.

7 Cooking
Use toothpick to achieve desired taste.

Single Oils

Grapefruit
Citrus X Paradisi

Application

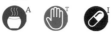

Chemical Constituents
d-Limonene
Nonanal
Nootketone

Other Uses
Anorexia, Bulimia, Dry Throat, Edema, Energy, Hangovers, Jet Lag, Lymphatic Congestion, Miscarriage Recovery, Obesity, Overeating

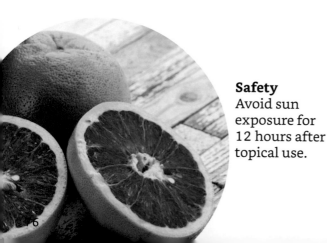

Safety
Avoid sun exposure for 12 hours after topical use.

Top *Uses*

1 Detox
Drink 1-3 drops in water.

2 Weight Loss
Apply 10 drops diluted with carrier oil over cellulite and fatty areas.

3 Smoking Addiction
Drink 1-3 drops in water after meals.

4 Antiviral Support
Apply 1-2 drops to bottoms of feet, or drink in water.

5 Appetite Suppressant
Diffuse several drops, or drink in water.

6 Gallbladder Stones
Drink 1-3 drops in water 3 times daily.

7 Food & Cooking
Use in smoothies, dressings, and sauces.

Helichrysum
Helichrysum Italicum

Application
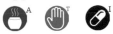

Chemical Constituents
Neryl Acetate
Italidione
y-curcumene

Other Uses
AIDS/HIV, Broken Blood Vessels, Bruises, Cuts, Earache, Fibroids, Gallbladder Infection, Hemorrhaging, Hernias, Herpes, Lymphatic Drainage, Nose Bleed, Sciatica, Staph Infection, Stretch Marks, Wrinkles

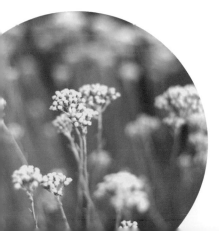

Top *Uses*

1 Tissue Repair
Apply neat or diluted to wounds.

2 Bleeding
Apply to clean wound to stop bleeding.

3 Eczema & Psoriasis
Apply 1-2 drops diluted to affected areas.

4 Shock
Diffuse 3-6 drops.

5 Tinnitus
Apply a drop behind ear.

6 Viral Infections
Take 1-2 drops in capsule, or diffuse.

7 Cholesterol
Take 1-3 drops in capsule, and apply to bottoms of feet.

Jasmine
Jasminum Grandiflorum

Application

A T I

Chemical Constituents
Benzyl Acetate
Phytol
Squalene

Other Uses
Apathy, Anxiety, Dry Skin, Insecurity, Labor & Delivery, Low Libido, Menstrual Camps, Nervous Tension, Nervousness, Ovulation, Stress

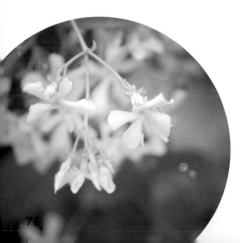

Top *Uses*

1 Depression & Self-Esteem Issues
Inhale 1-2 drops from cupped hands, or apply over heart.

2 Wrinkles & Fine Lines
Apply directly to desired areas.

3 Pink Eye
Apply carefully around affected eye, avoiding the eye itself.

4 Infertility
Apply to pulse points and reproductive reflex points.

5 Cramps & Spasms
Apply 1-2 drops to needed areas.

6 Lethargy & Fatigue
Inhale from cupped hands, or diffuse.

7 Sleep & Relaxation
Apply to bottoms of feet and temples.

Juniper Berry
Juniperus Communis

Application

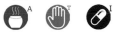

Chemical Constituents
a-pinene
B-caryophyllene
Bornyl Acetate

Other Uses
Acne, Anxiety, Bacteria, Bloating, Cellulite, Cystitis, Detoxifying, Fluid Retention, Heavy Legs, Jaundice, Menstrual Cramps, Mental Exhaustion, Stress, Ulcers, Viruses

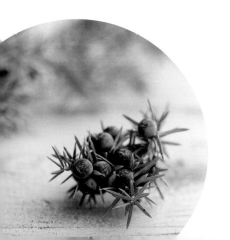

Top *Uses*

1 Kidney Detox & Infections
Rub 1-2 drops over kidneys, or take in capsule.

2 Diabetes
Take 1-2 drops in capsule daily.

3 Kidney Stones
Apply 1-2 drops over kidneys.

4 Urinary Tract Infection
Apply 1-2 drops over bladder.

5 High Cholesterol
Take 1-2 drops in capsule, or apply to bottoms of feet.

6 Tinnitus
Apply a drop behind affected ear.

7 Chronic Fatigue
Apply 1-2 drops to pulse points, or diffuse.

Single Oils

Kumquat
Fortunella Japonica

Application

Chemical Constituents
Limonene
Myrcene
a-Pinene

Other Uses
Antioxidant, Calming, Detoxification, Mental Stimulation, Revitalization, Shampoo & Conditioner Enhancer, Weight Loss

Safety
Avoid sun exposure for 12 hours after topical use.

Top *Uses*

1 Immune Support
Drink 1-3 drops in water, or apply to bottoms of feet.

2 Metabolism Boost
Drink 1-3 drops in water, or diffuse.

3 Mood Boost
Inhale 1-2 drops from cupped hands, or diffuse.

4 Energy
Drink 1-3 drops in water, or diffuse.

5 Household Cleaning
Use several drops in glass spray bottle with water.

6 Cardiovascular Health
Apply 1-2 drops to heart reflex points.

7 Nervous System Health
Apply 1-2 drops to bottoms of feet.

Lavender
Lavandula Angustifolia

Application

Chemical Constituents
Linalol
Linalyl Acetate
B-ocimene

Other Uses
Allergies, Bites, Blisters, Chicken Pox, Club Foot, Colic, Convulsions, Crying, Dandruff, Diaper Rash, Gangrene, Giardia, Impctigo, Insomnia, Poison Ivy & Oak, Seizures, Stings, Tachycardia, Teething Pain, Ticks

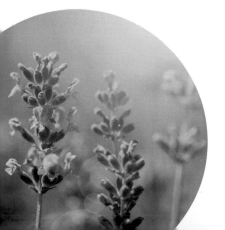

Top *Uses*

1 Stress & Anxiety
Apply 1-2 drops to temples, or diffuse.

2 Sleep
Apply 2 drops to bottoms of feet, or diffuse near bedside.

3 Skin Irritations & Burns
Apply 1-2 drops with carrier oil.

4 Allergies & Hay Fever
Put a drop under tongue for 30 seconds, then swallow with water.

5 Cuts, Blisters, & Scrapes
Apply diluted to affected areas.

6 Irritability
Apply 1-2 drops to pulse points.

7 Headaches & Migraines
Apply 1-2 drops to temples, and base of skull.

Lemon
Citrus Limon

Application

 A T I

Chemical Constituents
d-Limonene
Citral
Hexanol

Other Uses
Anxiety, Cold Sores, Colds, Concentration, Constipation, Depression, Disinfectant, Dysentery, Flu, Furniture Polish, Greasy Hair, High Blood Pressure, Kidney Stones, MRSA, Pancreatitis, Parasites, Tonsillitis

Safety
Avoid sun exposure for 12 hours after topical use.

Top *Uses*

1 Energy
Inhale 1-2 drops from cupped hands.

2 Detox
Drink 1-3 drops in water, or apply to bottoms of feet.

3 Permanent Marker
Rub several drops with clean rag.

4 Sore Throat
Take 1-2 drops with a spoonful of honey.

5 Increase Alkalinity
Drink 1-3 drops in water.

6 Household Cleaner
Use several drops with water in glass spray bottle.

7 Food & Cooking
Use in smoothies, juices, and sauces.

Lemongrass
Cymbopogon Flexuosus

Application

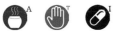

Chemical Constituents
Geranial
a-terpineol
Farnesol

Other Uses
Airborne Bacteria, Bladder Infection, Carpal Tunnel, Charley Horses, Connective Tissue Injury, Constipation, Frozen Shoulder, Lymphatic Drainage, Paralysis, Sprains, Urinary Tract Infection

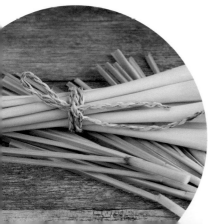

Safety
Possible skin sensitivity. Do not use internally more than 10 days in a row.

Top Uses

1 Thyroid Support (hypo & hyper)
Apply a drop diluted over thyroid.

2 High Cholesterol
Take 1-2 drops in capsule.

3 Ligament & Tendon Issues
Apply 1-2 drops diluted to painful areas.

4 Stomach Ulcers
Take 1 drop in capsule.

5 Immune Support
Apply 1-2 drops to bottoms of feet.

6 Lactose Intolerance
Take 1 drop in capsule.

7 Cooking
Use toothpick to achieve desired flavor.

Lime
Citrus Aurantifolia

Application

Chemical Constituents
d-Limonene
1,8 cineol
Geranial

Other Uses
Antiviral Support, Blood Pressure, Cellulite, Depression, Detox, Energy, Exhaustion, Fever, Gallstones, Gum Removal, Herpes, Memory, Water Purification

Safety
Avoid sun exposure for 12 hours after topical use.

Top *Uses*

1 Chronic Cough
Apply 2-4 drops over chest, mid-back, and lung reflex points.

2 Colds
Drink 1-3 drops in water, and diffuse.

3 Sore Throat
Gargle 2 drops with water.

4 Cold Sores
Apply 1 drop diluted to affected area.

5 Antioxidant
Drink 1-3 drops in water.

6 Bacterial Infections
Apply 1-2 drops with carrier oil to affected area.

7 Mental Clarity
Diffuse 3-6 drops, or inhale from cupped hands.

Litsea
Litsea Cubeba

Application

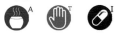 A T I

Chemical Constituents
Geranial
Neral
Limonene

Other Uses
Anxiety, Cold, Cough, Disinfectant, House-
hold Cleaning, Insect Repellent, Odors,
Perspiration, Sleep, Stress

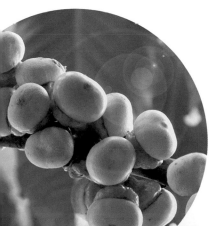

Safety
Possible skin
sensitivity.

1 Emotional Balance
*Diffuse several drops, or wear on scarf or
sleeve throughout the day.*

2 Mental Rejuvenation
Inhale 1-2 drops from cupped hands.

3 Postpartum Depression
Diffuse, or apply over heart area.

4 E. Coli
Apply 1-2 drops diluted to affected areas.

5 Internal Bacterial Infections
Drink 2-4 drops in water or in a capsule.

6 Aging
*Apply 1-2 drops in facial lotion to combat
age-promoting free radicals.*

7 Athlete's Foot
Apply 1-2 drops to clean feet.

Single Oils

Manuka
Leptospermum Scoparium

Application

Chemical Constituents
Eugenol
Eugenyl Acetate
B-caryophyllene

Other Uses
Athlete's Foot, Bronchitis, Catarrh, Contusions, Cough, Fungal Skin Infections, Head Lice, Influenza, Scabies, Skin Infection, Ulceration

Single Oils

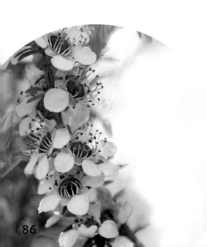

Safety
Possible skin sensitivity. Use with caution when pregnant.

Top *Uses*

1 Blemishes & Complexion
Add a couple drops to skincare products, or apply diluted to affected areas.

2 Hypertension
Apply 1-2 drops to pulse points, or diffuse.

3 Air Purification
Diffuse 4-8 drops.

4 Sleep
Graze pillows with a drop of oil, and diffuse near bedside.

5 Bronchial Infection
Inhale 1-2 drops from cupped hands, or diffuse.

6 Ringworm & Parasites
Apply 1-2 drops diluted to affected areas.

Marjoram
Origanum Majorana

Application
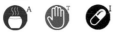

Chemical Constituents
a & y-terpinenes
a-terpineol
terpinen-4-ol

Other Uses
Arterial Vasodilator, Bruises, Colic, Constipation, Croup, Headache, Gastrointestinal Disorders, Insomnia, Menstrual Problems, Parkinson's, Prolapsed Mitral Valve, Ringworm, Sprains, Whiplash

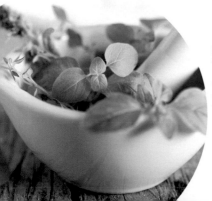

Safety
Use with caution during pregnancy.

Top *Uses*

1 Muscle Injury
Massage 2 drops with carrier oil into injured muscles.

2 Carpal Tunnel & Arthritis
Apply 1-2 drops neat to affected area.

3 High Blood Pressure
Apply 2 drops to bottoms of feet, or take in a capsule.

4 Irritable Bowel Syndrome
Take 1-2 drops in a capsule, or rub over abdomen.

5 Diverticulitis
Take 1-2 drops in a capsule.

6 Pancreatitis
Apply 1-2 drops neat over pancreas area.

7 Chronic Stress
Rub 1-2 drops onto back of neck.

Melaleuca
Melaleuca Alternifolia

Application

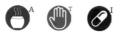

Chemical Constituents
a- & y-terpinenes
Terpinen-4-ol
a- & o-cadinenes

Other Uses
Aneurysm, Bacterial Infections, Cankers, Candida, Cavities, Cold Sores, Cuts, Dermatitis, Ear Infections, Fungal Infections, Hepatitis, Infected Wounds, MRSA, Nail Fungus, Pink Eye, Rubella, Thrush

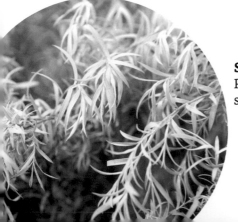

Safety
Possible skin sensitivity.

Top *Uses*

1 Rashes & Eczema
Apply 1-2 drops diluted to affected areas.

2 Dandruff
Add 2 drops to shampoo daily.

3 Athlete's Foot
Apply 1-2 drops neat to clean feet.

4 Acne & Blemishes
Apply a dab to affected areas.

5 Staph Infections
Take 1-2 drops in capsule.

6 Strep Throat & Tonsillitis
Gargle 2 drops with water, and rub 1-2 drops diluted to outside of throat.

7 Herpes
Apply 1 drop diluted to affected areas.

Melissa
Melissa Officinalis

Application

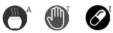 A   T   I

Chemical Constituents
Geranial
Germacrene-D
Linalol

Other Uses
Allergies, Anxiety, Blisters, Colds, Dysentery, Erysipelas, Hypertension, Nervousness, Sleep Disorders, Sterility, Viral Outbreak

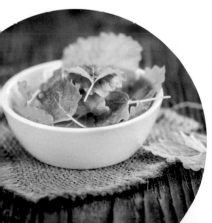

Safety
Dilute for sensitive skin.

Top *Uses*

1 Viral Infections
Take 1-2 drops in a capsule.

2 Cold Sores & Herpes
Apply a drop to affected areas.

3 Depression
Use thumb to hold a drop to the roof of the mouth.

4 Bronchitis, Asthma
Apply 1-2 drops diluted over chest.

5 Neurotonic
Apply a drop to the bottoms of feet.

6 Shock
Apply a drop diluted to back of neck, or diffuse.

7 Insomnia
Apply a drop to big toe, or use thumb to hold a drop to the roof of mouth.

Myrrh
Commiphora Myrrha

Application

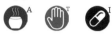

Chemical Constituents
Lindestrene
Methoxyfurogermacrene
Curzenone

Other Uses
Cancer, Chapped Skin, Congestion, Dysentery, Gum Bleeding, Hepatitis, Liver Cirrhosis, Scabies, Stretch Marks

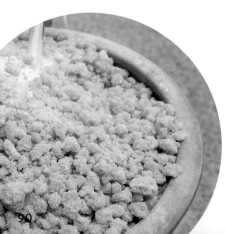

Safety
Use with caution during pregnancy.

Top *Uses*

1 **Wrinkles & Fine Lines**
Massage into needed areas as desired.

2 **Gum Disease & Issues**
Apply 1-2 drops to gums, or swish with water as mouth rinse.

3 **Thyroid Support**
Rub 1-2 drops over thyroid.

4 **Anxiety & Depression**
Inhale 1-2 drops from cupped hands, or diffuse.

5 **Mucus & Bronchitis**
Apply 1-2 drops to chest, or diffuse.

6 **Eczema & Skin Infections**
Apply 1-2 drops to affected areas.

7 **Nail Fungus**
Apply a drop to affected nails.

Neroli
Citrus Aurantium

Application
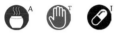

Chemical Constituents
Linalool
Geraniol
Limonene

Other Uses
Convalescence, Indigestion, Insomnia, Intestinal Cramping, Menopausal Anxiety, Sleep Disorders, Tension

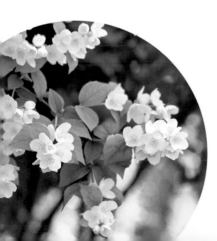

Top *Uses*

1 Scar Tissue & Stretch Marks
Massage a few drops with carrier oil into needed areas.

2 Perfume
Apply 1-2 drops to pulse points.

3 Cramps & Spasms
Apply neat to affected areas.

4 Emotional Exhaustion
Inhale from cupped hands, or diffuse.

5 Nervousness
Apply a drop to pulse points.

6 Depression
Wear as perfume, inhale from cupped hands, or diffuse.

7 Skin Regeneration
Apply generously to damaged or worn skin.

Oregano
Origanum Vulgare

Application

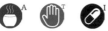

Chemical Constituents
Carvacrol
B-caryophyllene
Rosmaric Acid

Other Uses
Athlete's Foot, Calluses, Canker Sores, Carpal Tunnel, Control Issues, Ebola, Fungal Infections, Intestinal Parasites, MRSA, Nasal Polyps, Plague, Ringworm

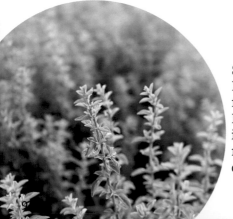

Safety
Heavily dilute for topical use. Do not use internally for more than 10 days in a row.

Top *Uses*

1 Bacterial & Viral Infection
Take 1-3 drops in a capsule for internal issues.

2 Warts
Apply directly to wart with toothpick, avoiding surrounding skin.

3 Candida & Staph Infection
Take 1-3 drops in a capsule.

4 Pneumonia & Whooping Cough
Diffuse 1-3 drops, sitting nearby the diffuser for several minutes. Also rub onto bottoms of feet.

5 Rheumatoid Arthritis
Massage 1 drop heavily diluted into affected area. Also take in a capsule.

6 Strep Throat & Tonsillitis
Gargle a drop in water. Also take 1-3 drops in capsule.

Patchouli
Pogostemon Cablin

Application

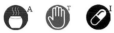

Chemical Constituents
a-bulesene
Patchoulol
Pathoulenone

Other Uses
Abscess, Cellulite, Chapped Skin, Depression, Dermatitis, Hemorrhoids, Hives, Irritability, Mastitis, Parasitic Skin Infection, PMS, Weeping Wounds

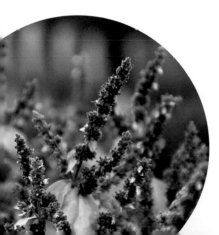

Top *Uses*

1 Diuretic
Apply 1-2 drops over lower abdomen.

2 Wrinkle Prevention
Add a drop to toner or moisturizer.

3 Shingles
Take 1-2 drops in capsule, or apply to bottoms of feet.

4 Dopamine Shortage
Diffuse 2-4 drops, or apply to pulse points.

5 Dandruff
Massage 1-2 drops into clean, dry scalp after showering.

6 Weight Loss
Take 1-2 drops with other weight loss essential oils in a capsule.

Single Oils

Peppermint
Menta Piperita

Application

Chemical Constituents
Menthol
a & B=pinenes
Germacrene-D

Other Uses
Alertness, Allergies, Autism, Burns, Cravings, Gastritis, Hangover, Hot Flashes, Hypothyroidism, Loss of Sense of Smell, Memory, Milk Supply (Decrease), Osteoporosis, Sciatica, Sinusitis, Typhoid

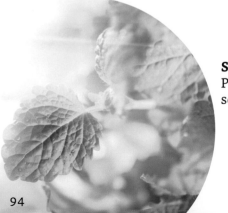

Safety
Possible skin sensitivity.

Top *Uses*

1 Headache & Migraine
Massage 1-2 drops into temples and base of skull, avoiding the eyes.

2 Digestive Upset
Drink 1-2 drops in water, or massage directly over stomach.

3 Asthma & Cough
Apply 2 drops with carrier oil over chest and lung reflex points, or diffuse.

4 Bad Breath
Lick a dab from your finger.

5 Low Energy & Mental Fog
Drink 1-2 drops in water, or diffuse.

6 Muscle & Joint Pain
Rub a drop diluted into affected areas.

7 Fevers
Apply 1-2 drops to back of neck.

Petitgrain
Citrus Aurantium

Application

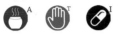

Chemical Constituents
Linalyl acetate
Linalool
Alpha-terpineol

Other Uses
Abdominal Cramps/Spasms, Aches, Acne, Convalescence, Depression, Hysteria, Infected Wounds, Nausea, Nervous Asthma, Oily Hair, Shock, Stress-Related Conditions, Tension

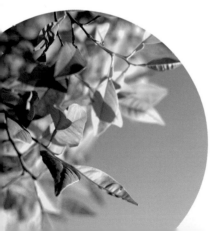

Safety
Use with caution during pregnancy.

Top *Uses*

1 Nervous & Muscular Spasms
Apply 1-2 drops to bottoms of feet, or to area of spasm.

2 Seizures
Apply 1-2 drops to bottoms of feet and back of neck.

3 Insomnia
Use a drop under tongue, or on pulse points. Also diffuse.

4 Irritability & Stress
Apply a drop behind ears, or wear as cologne on pulse points.

5 Bacterial Infections
Apply topically to affected area, or take 1-3 drops in a capsule.

6 Spastic Coughing
Apply 1-2 drops with carrier oil over chest and mid-back, or diffuse.

Red Mandarin
Citrus Reticulata

Application

Chemical Constituents
Limonene
Gamma-Terpinene

Other Uses
Household Cleaning, Intestinal Spasm, Irritability, Nervous Spasm, Sleeping Disorders, Stomachache, Stress

Safety
Avoid sun exposure for 12 hours after topical use.

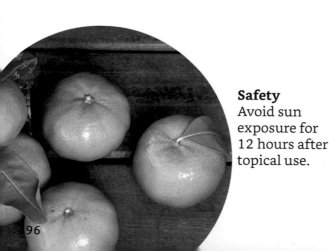

Top *Uses*

1 Skin Cleansing
Add a drop to facial cleanser.

2 Uplift & Energize
Inhale 1-2 drops from cupped hands, drink in water, or diffuse.

3 Digestive Conditions & IBS
Drink 1-3 drops in water.

4 Cellulite
Massage several drops with carrier oil over cellulite.

5 Antioxidant
Drink 1-3 drops in water, or apply over lymph nodes.

6 Constipation
Rub 2-4 drops clockwise over abdomen.

7 Convalescence
Diffuse and wear on pulse points.

Single Oils

Roman Chamomile
Anthemis Nobilis

Application
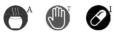

Chemical Constituents
Isobutyl
a- & B-pinenes
Pinocarvone

Other Uses
Allergies, Anorexia, Bee/Hornet Stings, Club Foot, Dysentery, Hyperactivity, Menopause, Muscle Spasms, Neuralgia, Rashes, Shock, Sore Nipples

Top *Uses*

1 Sleep & Insomnia
Apply 1-2 drops to temples and wrists, or diffuse next to bedside.

2 Panic Attacks
Carry on person and breathe a drop deeply from cupped hands as needed.

3 Diaper Rash
Apply 1 drop heavily diluted with carrier oil to baby skin.

4 Crying
Add a drop to front of shirt or sleeve, or diffuse.

5 PMS & Cramps
Apply a drop over abdomen.

6 Parasites & Worms
Apply 1-2 drops over abdomen, and take in a capsule.

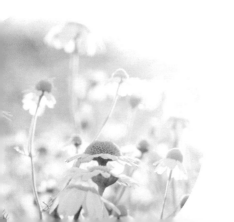

Rose
Rosa Damascena

Application

 A   T   I

Chemical Constituents
Citronellol
Stearoptene
Nonadecane

Other Uses
Anxiety, Astringent, Dysmenorrhea, Endo-
metriosis, Grief, Facial Redness, Impotency,
Infertility, Irregular Ovulation, Menstrual
Cramping, Phobias

Safety
Use with
caution during
pregnancy.

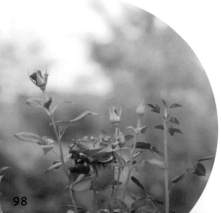

Top *Uses*

1 Aging Skin
*Add a drop to toner or moisturizer, or
apply with carrier oil over fine lines, wrinkles, and age spots.*

2 Low Libido
*Apply 1-2 drops to pulse points, or to
reproductive reflex points.*

3 Scar Tissue
Massage into scar tissue 3 times daily.

4 Self-Esteem & Depression
Apply 1-2 drops over heart, or diffuse.

5 Aphrodisiac
*Diffuse a few drops, or wear on pulse
points.*

6 Poison Ivy/Oak
Apply 1-2 drops diluted to irritated areas.

Rosemary
Rosmarinus Officinalis

Application
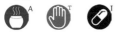

Chemical Constituents
1, 8 Cineol
a-pinene
Camphor

Other Uses
Alcohol Addiction, Adenitis, Arthritis, Bell's Palsy, Cellulite, Club Foot, Constipation, Headaches, Kidney Infection, Lice, Muscular Dystrophy, Osteoarthritis, Schmidt's Syndrome, Sinusitis

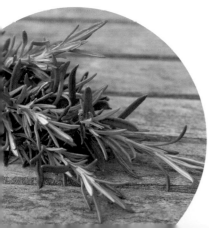

Safety
Avoid during pregnancy, if epileptic, or with high blood pressure.

Top *Uses*

1 Chronic Cough
Apply 2-4 drops to lung reflex points or diluted over chest, or diffuse.

2 Mental & Adrenal Fatigue
Inhale 1-2 drops from cupped hands, or take in a capsule.

3 Focus & Memory Issues
Apply a drop over forehead, or diffuse.

4 Cold & Flu
Apply 1-2 drops diluted over chest.

5 Low Blood Pressure
Massage with carrier oil into legs and on bottoms of feet.

6 Jet Lag
Apply 1-2 drops to temples after flying.

7 Hair Loss.
Work 2 drops into scalp before washing.

Sandalwood
Santalum Album

Application

Chemical Constituents
a & B-santalols
a- & B-santalenes
Norticycloekasantalic Acid

Other Uses
Aphrodisiac, Back Pain, Blemishes, Calming, Cartilage Repair, Coma, Dry Skin/Scalp, Exhaustion, Hiccups, Laryngitis, Lou Gehrig's Disease, Moles, Multiple Sclerosis, UV Radiation, Yoga

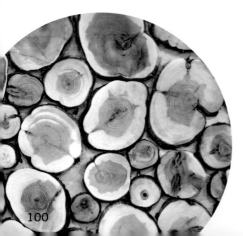

Top *Uses*

1 Rashes & Skin Conditions
Apply 1-2 drops with carrier oil to affected areas.

2 Cancer & Tumors
Take 1-2 drops in capsule, apply diluted to affected area, or diffuse.

3 Meditation
Apply a drop to temples during meditation.

4 Low Testosterone
Take 1-2 drops in a capsule, or apply to pulse points and lower abdomen.

5 Scars
Massage 1-2 drops into scars often.

6 Alzheimer's Disease
Apply 1-2 drops to base of skull, or take 1-2 drops in capsule daily.

Siberian Fir
Abies Sibirica

Application

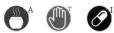

Chemical Constituents
Bornyl Acetate
Terpinyl Acetate
Camphene

Other Uses
Anxiety, Bronchitis, Catarrh, Fever, Sinusitis, Sluggish Nerves, Tension, Urinary Infection

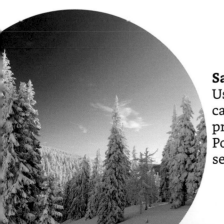

Safety
Use with caution during pregnancy. Possible skin sensitivity.

Top *Uses*

1 Asthma
Apply 1-2 drops with carrier oil over chest or to lung reflex points.

2 Immune Stimulant
Apply 1-2 drops to bottoms of feet.

3 Dry Cough, Cold, & Flu
Inhale 1-2 drops from cupped hands, or apply with carrier oil over chest.

4 Muscle Cramps & Spasms
Massage several drops with carrier oil into affected areas.

5 Emotional Overwhelm
Inhale 1-2 drops from cupped hands.

6 Rheumatism
Apply 1-2 drops neat to affected areas.

7 Mucus
Apply 1-2 drops to throat and chest.

Spearmint
Mentha Spicata

Application
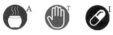 A   T   I

Chemical Constituents
l-carvone
l-limonene
Carveol

Other Uses
Acne, Bronchitis, Headaches, Focus, Migraines, Nervous Fatigue, Respiratory Infection, Sores, Scars

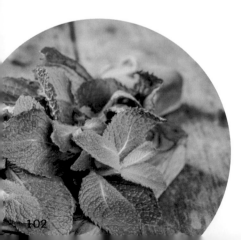

Top *Uses*

1 Indigestion
Drink 1-2 drops in water or in a capsule.

2 Colic
Apply a drop heavily diluted to baby's stomach.

3 Nausea
Inhale 1-2 drops from cupped hands, or rub over stomach.

4 Muscle Aches
Massage 1-2 drops diluted over achy muscles.

5 Bad Breath
Swish 1-2 drops in water as a mouthwash.

6 Heavy Menstruation
Apply 1-2 drops over back of neck and abdomen, or diffuse.

Spikenard
Nardostachys Jatamansi

Application
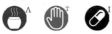

Chemical Constituents
Jatamansone
Nardol
a-Selinene

Other Uses
Constipation, Depression, Estrogen Imbalance, Fungal Issues, Mental Fatigue, Pinkeye, PMS Cramping, Progesterone Imbalance, Uterus & Ovaries Detox

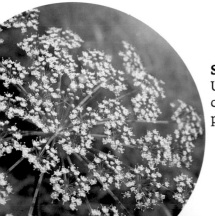

Safety
Use with caution during pregnancy.

Top *Uses*

1 Chronic Fatigue Syndrome
Apply 1-2 drops to adrenals and pulse points, or take in a capsule.

2 Insomnia
Put a drop under the tongue, or take in a capsule.

3 Toenail Fungus
Apply neat to affected toenail often.

4 Digestive Inflammation
Take 1-2 drops in a capsule.

5 Pancreatitis
Apply 1-2 drops neat over pancreas.

6 Immune Stimulant
Apply 1-2 drops to bottoms of feet.

7 Hair Loss
Add 2 drops to shampoo, and take 1-2 drops in a capsule.

Single Oils

Tangerine
Citrus Reticulata

Application

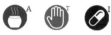

Chemical Constituents
d-limonene
B-carotene
Linalol

Other Uses
Anxious Feelings, Chronic Fatigue, Circulation, Detox, Digestive Problems, Muscle Aches, Muscle Spasms, Parasites, Water Retention

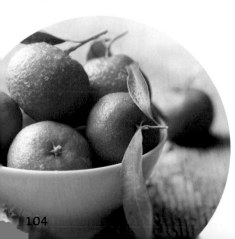

Safety
Avoid sun exposure for 12 hours after topical use.

Top *Uses*

1 Stress-Induced Insomnia
Inhale 1-2 drops during stressfull times of the day. Use a drop under the tongue before bedtime.

2 Cellulite
Massage several drops with carrier oil into cellulite areas.

3 Nervous Exhaustion
Diffuse 4-8 drops, or wear a drop on pulse points.

4 Congestion
Rub 2-4 drops over chest and mid-back.

5 Discouragement
Inhale 1-2 drops from cupped hands. Also add 1-3 drops to water.

6 Flatulence & Constipation
Rub 1-2 drops clockwise over stomach, or drink with water.

Thyme
Thymus Vulgaris

Application

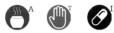 A   T   I

Chemical Constituents
Thymol
p-cymene
Linalol

Other Uses
Antioxidant, Asthma, Bites/Stings, Blood Clots, Croup, Eczema/Dermatitis, Fragile Hair, Fungal Infections, Greasy Hair, Hair Loss, Laryngitis, Mold, Numbness, Parasites, Prostatitis, Tendinitis, Tuberculosis

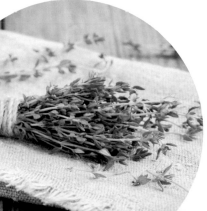

Safety
Possible skin sensitivity. Use with caution during pregnancy or with high blood pressure.

Top *Uses*

1 Bacterial Infection
Take 1-2 drops in a capsule, or apply to bottoms of feet.

2 Mononucleosis
Take 2 drops in a capsule 3 times daily. Also apply to bottoms of feet.

3 Cough, Cold, & Flu
Diffuse 1-2 drops, and take in a capsule.

4 Bronchitis
Apply 1-2 drops heavily diluted over chest and lung reflex points.

5 Skin Infections
Apply a drop heavily diluted to affected area.

6 Chronic Fatigue
Take 1-2 drops in a capsule, or apply heavily diluted over adrenal glands. Also use one drop in a hot bath.

Single Oils

Vetiver
Vetiveria Zizanioides

Application

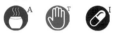

Chemical Constituents
Isovalencenol
a- & B-vetivones
Vitivene

Other Uses
Breast Enlargement, Depression, Irritability, Learning Difficulties, Memory Retention, Muscular Pain, Nerve Issues, Nervous Tension, PMS, Postpartum Depression, Restlessness, Termites, Workaholism

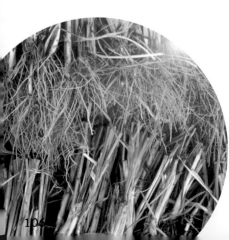

Top *Uses*

1 ADD/ADHD
Apply 1-2 drops behind ears and on the back of the neck.

2 Sleep & Insomnia
Apply 1-2 drops along spine.

3 Skin Irritation
Apply 1-2 drops with carrier oil to affected area.

4 Neuropathy
Apply 1-2 drops to bottoms of feet, or along spine.

5 Balance Issues
Apply 1-2 drops behind ears.

6 Stress-Related Menstrual Issues
Apply 1-2 drops to lower abdomen.

7 PTSD & Anxiety
Apply 1-2 drops behind ears, or diffuse.

White Fir
Abies Alba

Application
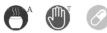 A   T   I

Chemical Constituents
l-limonene
a-pinene
Bornyle Acetate

Other Uses
Bruising, Bursitis, Circulation, Frozen Shoulder, Furniture Polish, Joint Pain, Muscle Fatigue, Sinusitis, Stress, Urinary Infection

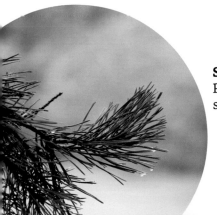

Safety
Possible skin sensitivity.

Top *Uses*

1 Bronchitis & Cough
Apply 2-4 drops over chest and mid-back, or diffuse.

2 Asthma
Apply 1-2 drops to lung reflex points, and inhale from cupped hands.

3 Muscle Aches & Pain
Massage 1-2 drops with carrier oil into affected areas.

4 Cartilage Inflammation
Apply 1-2 drops neat to affected areas.

5 Sprains
Massage 1-2 drops with carrier oil into affected areas.

6 Airborne Pathogens
Diffuse 5-10 drops.

Single Oils

Wild Orange
Citrus Sinensis

Single Oils

Application

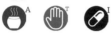

Chemical Constituents
d-Limonene
B-carotene
Citral

Other Uses
Cellulite, Colds, Creativity, Depression, Detox, Fear, Fluid Retention, Heart Palpitations, Insomnia, Menopause, Nervousness, Scurvy, Sluggish Digestion, Withdrawal Issues

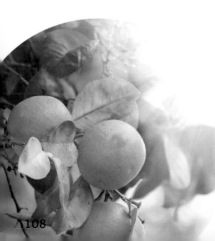

Safety
Avoid sun exposure for 12 hours after topical use.

Top *Uses*

1 Energy
Drink 1-3 drops in water, or inhale from cupped hands.

2 Cheering & Mood Enhancer
Inhale 1-2 drops from cupped hands, or diffuse.

3 Anxiety & Depression
Inhale 1-2 drops from cupped hands, or diffuse 5-10 drops.

4 Immune Support
Gargle 2 drops with water, or apply to bottoms of feet.

5 Sleep Issues
Put a drop under the tongue before bed.

6 Smoothies, Dressings, & Sauces
Add according to taste.

Wintergreen
Gaultheria Procumbens

Application
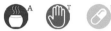

Chemical Constituents
Methyl Salicylate
Salicylic Acid

Other Uses
Bone Spurs, Cartilage Injury, Circulation, Muscle Development, Rheumatism

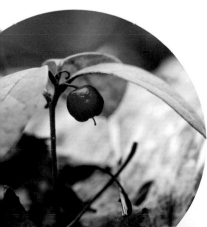

Safety
Potential skin sensitivity.

Top *Uses*

1 Muscle Pain & Inflammation
Massage 1-2 drops with carrier oil into affected areas.

2 Arthritis & Gout
Massage 1-2 drops into inflamed joints, diluting if needed.

3 Broken Bones
Apply 1-2 drops gently over injury, avoiding open wounds.

4 Frozen Shoulder & Rotator Cuff
Massage 1-2 drops with carrier oil into affected area.

5 Teeth Whitening
Brush with a drop of oil and baking soda.

6 Dandruff
Add a drop to shampoo, or massage 1-2 drops directly into scalp before shampooing.

Yarrow
Achillea Millefolium

Application

 A   T   I

Chemical Constituents
Azulene
Caryophyllene
Pinene

Other Uses
Congestion, Detox, Excess Sodium, Digestive Discomfort, Flatulence, Gallbladder Pain, Headache, Heart Attack, Inflammation, Metabolism, Muscle Spasms, PMS, Weight Loss

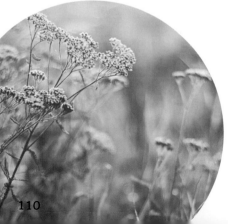

Safety
Can irritate sensitive skin. Avoid long-term use in high doses.

Top *Uses*

1 Rheumatism & Arthritis
Massage 1-2 drops with carrier oil into affected area.

2 Muscle Injury & Cramps
Massage 1-2 drops into affected area, diluting if needed.

3 Scars
Massage 1-2 drops into scar tissue.

4 Acne
Add a drop to toner or facial cleanser.

5 Varicose Veins
Apply 1-2 drops neat to affected areas.

6 Hemorrhoids
Apply 1-2 drops heavily diluted to affected area.

7 Eczema & Skin Irritation
Apply 1-2 drops diluted to affected area.

Ylang Ylang
Cananga Odorata

Application

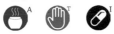

Chemical Constituents
B-caryophylle
Benzyl Acetate & Benzoate
Linalol

Other Uses
Anxiety, Arterial Hypertension, Balance Issues, Chronic Fatigue, Circulation, Depression, Diabetes, Exhaustion, Hair Loss, Hypertension, Insomnia, Intestinal Spasms, Tachycardia

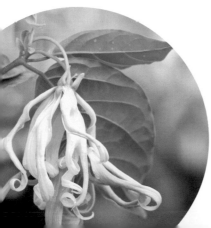

Safety
Dilute for highly sensitive skin.

Top *Uses*

1 Hormone Balance
Apply 1-2 drops to wrists and behind ears.

2 Low Libido
Apply 1-2 drops to pulse points and reproductive reflex points. Diffuse 4-8 drops during intimacy, or use in massage.

3 High Blood Pressure
Apply 2 drops to bottoms of feet, and take in capsule daily.

4 Infertility
Massage 1-2 drops over abdomen and reproductive reflex points.

5 Heart Palpitations
Apply 1-2 drops over heart, and diffuse.

6 Oily Skin
Add a drop to toner or facial moisturizer, or take 1-2 drops in a capsule daily.

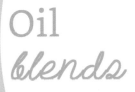

Section 5

Oil
blends

Anti-Aging Blend

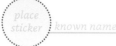

 known name

Application

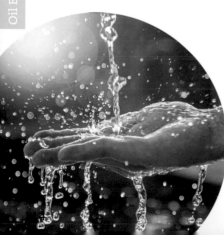

Main Ingredients
Frankincense, Sandalwood, Lavender, Myrrh, Helichrysum, Rose

Other Uses
Aging, Blisters, Chapped Skin, Cuts, Dry Skin, Eczema, Hyper-pigmentation, Psoriasis, Sun Burns

Oil Blends

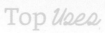

1 Wrinkles & Fine Lines
Apply to desired areas morning and night.

2 Age Spots
Apply to affected areas 3 times daily.

3 Scarring
Massage for 30 seconds into scar tissue 2-3 times a day until desired appearance.

4 Skin Cancer
Apply neat to affected area 3x/day.

5 Skin Discoloration
Apply to affected areas 3 times daily.

6 Meditation
Apply to pulse points during meditation.

7 Bleeding
Apply neat to stop minor bleeding.

Cellular Complex

place sticker known name

Application

A T I

Main Ingredients

Frankincense, Wild Orange, Lemongrass, Thyme, Summer Savory, Clove, Niaouli

Other Uses

Addictions, Blood Clots, Candida, Cataracts, Fever, Herpes Simplex, Hodgkin's Disease, Glaucoma, Gingivitis, Lipoma, Lupus, Lyme

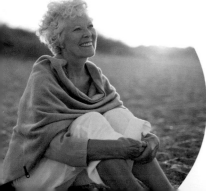

Safety

Can irritate sensitive skin. Use with caution during pregnancy.

Top *Uses*

1 Thyroid (hypo, Hashimoto's)
Apply diluted over thyroid or to thyroid reflex point, or take 1-2 drops in capsule.

2 Toothache
Apply directly to problematic tooth.

3 Smoking Addiction
Rub onto bottom of big toe.

4 Immune Support
Take 1-2 drops in a capsule.

5 Antioxidant
Take 1-2 drops in a capsule, or use in cooking.

6 Liver Detox
Rub over liver, or on liver reflex point.

7 Rheumatoid Arthritis
Massage diluted into affected area.

Oil Blends

115

Cleansing Blend

 known name _____

Application

Main Ingredients
Lime, Lemon, Siberian Fir, Citronella, Melaleuca, Cilantro

Other Uses
Airborne Bacteria & Viruses, Boils, Household Cleaning, Insect Repellent, Mice Repellent, Skin Ulcers

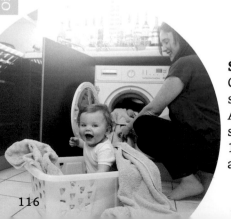

Safety
Can irritate sensitive skin. Avoid direct sun exposure 12 hours after application.

Oil Blends

Top *Uses*

1 Air Freshener
Add 10 drops to glass spray bottle with water. Spray as needed.

2 Foot Odors
Apply neat to feet. Spray inside shoes.

3 Laundry
Add 4-5 drops to detergent.

4 Disinfectant
Add 20 drops to glass spray bottle with water and 1 Tbs rubbing alcohol.

5 Deodorant
Apply 1-2 drops with carrier oil to armpits.

6 Mildew
Use several drops with a clean sponge.

7 Bites & Stings
Apply 1 drop neat to bite or sting.

Comforting Blend

place sticker / *known name* _____

Application

 A   T   I

Main Ingredients

Frankincense, Ylang Ylang, Patchouli, Laudanum, Sandalwood, Rose, Osmanthus

Other Uses

Anger, Brain Health, Bladder Infection, Emotional Processing, Heart Health, Resentment

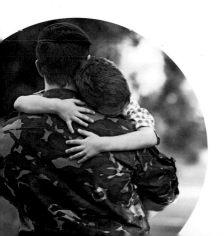

Top *Uses*

1 Grief, Sorrow, Despair
Apply 1-2 drops over heart, or diffuse.

2 Hormone Balance
Apply 1-2 drops to pulse points before bed.

3 Self-Esteem
Inhale from cupped hands, or diffuse during meditation.

4 Perfume
Wear on pulse points for a floral aroma.

5 Anti-Aging
Apply 1-2 drops with carrier oil to wrinkles, sun spots, and fine lines.

6 Nightmares
Diffuse 3-6 drops next to bedside.

7 Rheumatoid Arthritis
Massage diluted into affected area.

Detoxification Blend

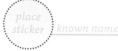
known name _____

Application

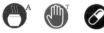
A T I

Main Ingredients
Tangerine, Geranium, Rosemary, Juniper Berry, Cilantro

Other Uses
Hangover, Hormone Balance, Gallbladder Detox, Urinary Infection, Weight Loss

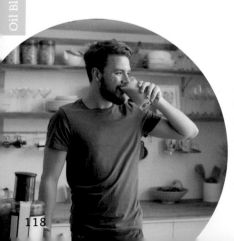

Safety
Can irritate sensitive skin. Avoid sun exposure for 12 hours after topical use.

Top *Uses*

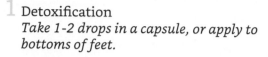

1 Detoxification
Take 1-2 drops in a capsule, or apply to bottoms of feet.

2 Allergies
Apply 1-2 drops to bottoms of feet, or diffuse.

3 Smoking Cravings
Rub onto bottom of big toe, or drink 1-3 drops in water after meals.

4 Liver & Kidney Support
Massage 1-2 drops over liver or kidneys.

5 Antioxidant
Take 1-2 drops in a capsule.

6 Heavy Metal Detox
Apply 1-2 drops to bottoms of feet.

7 Adrenal Fatigue
Massage 1-2 drops over lower back.

Digestive Blend

place sticker _____ known name _____

Application

 A   🖐 T   💊 I

Main Ingredients

Peppermint, Ginger, Caraway, Coriander, Anise, Tarragon

Other Uses

Abdominal Cramps, Acid Reflux, Colitis, Crohn's Disease, Gastritis, Heartburn, Morning Sickness, Motion Sickness, Parasites, Sinusitis

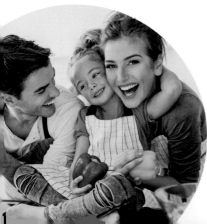

Safety

Can irritate sensitive skin. Use with caution during pregnancy.

Top *Uses*

1 Stomach Upset
Drink 1-2 drops in water, or take in a capsule.

2 Gas & Bloating
Massage 1-2 drops over stomach, or take in a capsule.

3 Diarrhea & Constipation
Massage 1-2 drops over stomach, or take in a capsule.

4 Irritable Bowel Syndrome
Massage 1-2 drops over stomach, or take in a capsule.

5 Food Poisoning
Drink 1-2 drops in water, or take in a capsule.

6 Nausea
Put a drop under the tongue, or rub over stomach.

Encouraging Blend

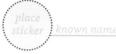

place sticker *known name*

Application

A   T   I

Main Ingredients
Clementine, Peppermint, Coriander, Basil, Melissa, Rosemary

Other Uses
Asthma, Confusion, Creativity, Fatigue, Loneliness, Overwhelm, Uncertainty

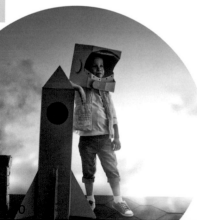

Safety
Can irritate sensitive skin. Use with caution during pregnancy.

Top *Uses*

1 Discouragement, Low Confidence, Low Motivation
Inhale 1-2 drops from cupped hands, or diffuse.

2 Detox
Apply 1-2 drops to bottoms of feet, or massage over endocrine organs.

3 Adrenal Fatigue
Massage 1-2 drops with carrier oil over lower back.

4 Flatulence
Rub 1-2 drops with carrier oil over stomach.

5 Depression
Diffuse 5-10 drops, or rub 1-2 drops onto temples.

6 Respiratory Issues
Apply 1-2 drops over chest, or diffuse.

Focus Blend

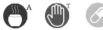
known name

Application

A   T   I

Main Ingredients
Amyris, Patchouli, Frankincense, Lime, Ylang Ylang, Sandalwood, Chamomile

Other Uses
Alzheimer's, Emotional Balance, Hormone Balance, Memory, Parkinson's, Relaxation, Sleep

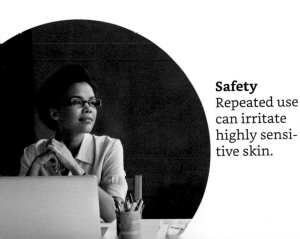

Safety
Repeated use can irritate highly sensitive skin.

1 ADD & ADHD
Apply to back of neck and behind ears.

2 Focus & Concentration
Apply to back of neck and behind ears.

3 Anxiety
Apply to pulse points, or inhale from cupped hands.

4 Hyperactivity
Apply to pulse points, or inhale from cupped hands.

5 Scizures
Apply to bottoms of feet and back of neck.

6 Skin Irritations
Apply with carrier oil to affected areas.

7 Sedative
Apply to pulse points or bottoms of feet.

Oil Blends

121

Grounding Blend

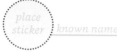

place sticker _known name_

Application

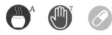

Main Ingredients
Spruce, Ho Wood, Frankincense, Blue Tansy, Blue Chamomile

Other Uses
Anger, Back Pain, Brain Integration, Bursitis, Comas, Confusion, Convulsions, Diabetic Sores, Grief, Herniated Discs, Hyperactivity, Lou Gehrig's Disease, Parkinson's Disease, Tranquility

Top Uses

1 Emotional Grounding
Inhale 1-2 drops from cupped hands, or apply to bottoms of feet daily.

2 Focus & Concentration
Apply 1-2 drops to temples and pulse points, or diffuse.

3 Stress & Anxiety
Apply 1-2 drops to pulse points and temples, or to bottoms of feet.

4 Meditation
Apply 1-2 drops to wrists and temples.

5 Neurological Issues
Apply 1-2 drops to bottoms of feet.

6 Stress-Induced Inflammation
Inhale 1-2 drops from cupped hands, apply to bottoms of feet, or diffuse.

7 Balance
Apply 1-2 drops behind ears.

Holiday Blend

place sticker *known name* _____

Application

A T I

Main Ingredients
Siberian Fir, Orange, Clove, Cinnamon, Douglas Fir, Vanilla, Nutmeg

Other Uses
Arthritis, Blood Sugar Balance, Muscle Tension, Respiratory Conditions

Safety
Can irritate sensitive skin.

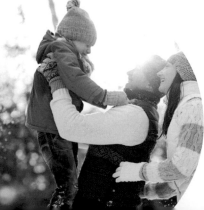

Top *Uses*

1 Joyful Feelings
Diffuse 5-10 drops, or inhale 1-2 drops from cupped hands.

2 Cover Burnt Food Smell
Diffuse 5-10 drops.

3 Stress & Tension
Apply 1-2 drops with carrier oil to pulse points.

4 Family Contention
Diffuse 5-10 drops.

5 Cold & Flu
Apply 1-2 drops to bottoms of feet.

6 Airborne Pathogens
Diffuse 5-10 drops.

Oil Blends

Hopeful Blend

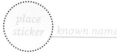
place sticker *known name*

Application

Main Ingredients
Bergamot*, Ylang Ylang, Frankincense, Vanilla

Other Uses
Addictions, Alzheimer's, Appetite Loss, Autism, Discouragement, Parkinson's, Self-Worth Issues

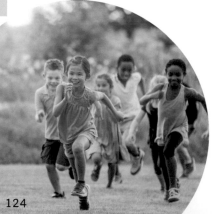

Safety
*FCF Bergamot does not cause photo sensitivity.

Top *Uses*

1 Emotional Trauma
Apply to pulse points, and inhale from cupped hands.

2 Grief & Trust Issues
Apply to pulse points, and inhale from cupped hands.

3 Hormone Balance
Apply to wrists and bottoms of feet.

4 Perfume
Apply 1-2 drops to pulse points.

5 Adrenal Fatigue
Apply to neck and lower back.

6 Stress
Apply to temples, and inhale from cupped hands.

7 Focus & Concentration
Apply to temples.

Inspiring Blend

Application

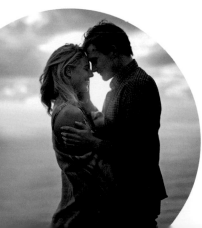

Main Ingredients
Cardamom, Cinnamon, Ginger, Sandalwood, Jasmine

Other Uses
Depression, Hormone Balance, Menopause, PMS Discomfort, Slow Bowel Movements

Safety
Can irritate sensitive skin. Avoid topical use during pregnancy.

Top Uses

1 Apathy & Boredom
Inhale 1-2 drops from cupped hands, or diffuse.

2 Low Sex Drive
Apply 1-2 drops with carrier oil to pulse points, or use diluted in massage.

3 Digestive Issues
Apply 1-2 drops to stomach reflex points, or apply diluted over stomach.

4 Aphrodisiac
Apply 1-2 drops to pulse points.

5 Slow Digestion
Apply 1-2 drops with carrier oil over stomach.

6 Lack of Creativity
Diffuse 5-10 drops.

Oil Blends

125

Invigorating Blend

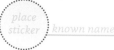
known name

Application

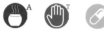

Main Ingredients
Orange, Lemon, Grapefruit, Mandarin, Bergamot, Clementine, Vanilla

Other Uses
Air Freshener, Household Cleaning, Eating Disorders, Laundry Freshener, Low Appetite, Mastitis

Safety
Avoid sun exposure for 12 hours after topical use.

Top _Uses_

1 Lack of Creativity & Inspiration
Inhale 2 drops from cupped hands, or diffuse.

2 Low Energy
Apply 2 drops to pulse points, or diffuse.

3 Morning Moodiness
Diffuse 5-10 drops next to bedside in the morning, or inhale from cupped hands.

4 Lymphatic Drainage
Apply 3-4 drops to bottoms of feet.

5 Stress & Anxiety
Inhale 2 drops from cupped hands, or apply to pulse points.

6 Depression & Moodiness
Inhale 2 drops from cupped hands, or diffuse 5-10 drops.

Joyful Blend

place sticker _known name_

Application

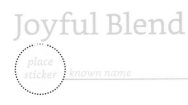^A ^T ^I

Main Ingredients

Lavandin, Lavender, Sandalwood, Tangerine, Melissa, Ylang Ylang, Osmanthus, Lemon Myrtle

Other Uses

Cushing's Syndrome, Lethargy, Postpartum Depression, Sadness, Shock, Weight Loss

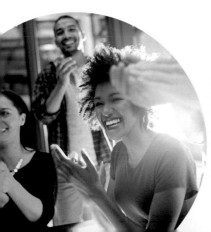

Safety

Can irritate sensitive skin. Avoid sun exposure for 12 hours after topical use.

Top *Uses*

1 **Depression**
Carry on your person, and inhale 1-2 drops from cupped hands as needed.

2 **Stress & Anxiety**
Diffuse 4-8 drops, or inhale 1-2 drops from cupped hands.

3 **Abuse Recovery**
Apply 1-2 drops to back of neck and over heart.

4 **Grief & Sorrow**
Apply 1-2 drops to pulse points, or diffuse.

5 **Poison Oak/Ivy**
Apply 1-2 drops with carrier oil to affected areas.

6 **Lupus & Fibromyalgia**
Inhale 1-2 drops from cupped hands, and apply diluted to inflamed areas.

Oil Blends

127

Massage Blend

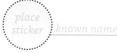
place sticker *known name*

Application

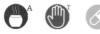

Main Ingredients

Cypress, Peppermint, Marjoram, Basil, Grapefruit, Lavender

Other Uses

Arthritis, Circulation, Ligament Damage, Muscular Dystrophy, Relaxation, Tension

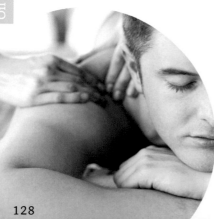

Safety
Can irritate sensitive skin. Use with caution during pregnancy.

Top *Uses*

1 Muscle Tension & Aches
Massage 2-4 drops with carrier oil into tight muscles.

2 Adrenal Fatigue & Lethargy
Apply 1-2 drops to lower back.

3 Back, Neck, & Shoulder Pain
Massage 2-4 drops with carrier oil into affected muscles, or add to hot bath.

4 Post-Work Stress
Massage 2 drops into back of neck to relieve stress from work.

5 Neuropathy
Apply 1-2 drops to bottoms of feet.

6 High Blood Pressure
Apply 1-2 drops to bottoms of feet.

7 Headache
Apply 1-2 drops to temples, avoiding eyes.

Metabolic Blend

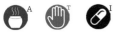

known name _____

Application

A T I

Main Ingredients
Grapefruit, Lemon, Ginger, Peppermint, Cinnamon

Other Uses
Colds, Congestion, Detox, Energy, Food Addiction, Gallbladder Stones, High Cholesterol, Lymphatic Stimulation, Obesity, Over-Eating

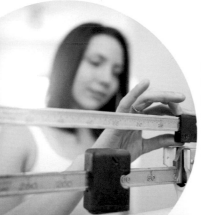

Safety
Can irritate sensitive skin. Use with caution during pregnancy.

Top *Uses*

1 Weight Loss
Take 2-4 drops in capsule or drink in water.

2 Appetite Control
Drink 2-4 drops in water throughout the day, or diffuse.

3 Blood Sugar Regulation
Take 1-2 drops in water or in a capsule.

4 Cellulite & Visceral Fat
Massage several drops with carrier oil into needed areas.

5 Antioxidant
Take 1-2 drops in a capsule.

6 Eating Disorders
Take a drop under the tongue, or diffuse 4-8 drops.

Oil Blends

Outdoor Blend

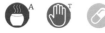

known name

Application

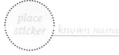

Main Ingredients

Catnip, Skimmia Laureola, Amyris, Balsam, Orange, White Fir, Eucalyptus, African Sandalwood, Genet, Rose

Other Uses

Ants, Mites, Termites, Tics

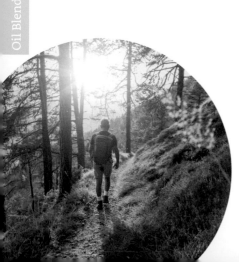

Top *Uses*

1 Insect Repellent
Apply directly to exposed skin, and diffuse if possible

2 Fly Infestation
Diffuse 10 drops, or apply lightly over clothing.

3 Energetic Toxicity
Use 1-3 drops during meditation, journaling, or prayer.

Protective Blend

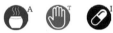
place sticker known name _____

Application

A T I

Main Ingredients
Orange, Clove, Cinnamon, Rosemary, Eucalyptus

Other Uses
Autoimmune Disorders, Cough, Germs, Household Cleaning, Hypoglycemia, Laundry Booster, Mold, Pneumonia, Staph Infection, Strep Throat, Warts

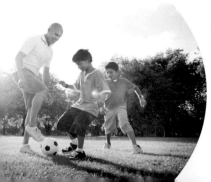

Safety
Can irritate sensitive skin. Use with caution during pregnancy.

Top Uses

1 Immune Support
Take 1-2 drops in capsule as daily supplement, or apply to bottoms of feet.

2 Colds & Flu
Apply 1-2 drops to bottoms of feet, and take with water or in a capsule.

3 Airborne Viruses
Diffuse 5-10 drops.

4 Mouthwash
Rinse mouth with 2 drops and water.

5 Cold Sores
Apply a drop with carrier oil to needed areas.

6 MRSA
Apply 1-2 drops diluted to affected areas.

7 Gum Disease & Cavities
Rinse mouth with 2 drops and water.

Oil Blends

Reassuring Blend

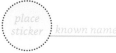

place sticker ___known name___

Application

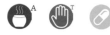 A T I

Main Ingredients

Vetiver, Lavender, Ylang Ylang, Frankincense, Marjoram, Spearmint, Labdanum

Other Uses

Addictive Personality, Postpartum Recovery, Social Anxiety

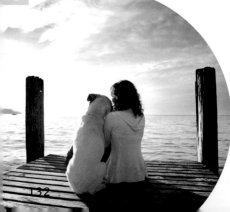

Safety

Use with caution during beginning of pregnancy.

Top *Uses*

1 Fear & Insecurity
Apply 1-2 drops over temples or chest.

2 Worry
Inhale 1-2 drops from cupped hands.

3 Restlessness & Irritability
Apply 1-2 drops to temples or bottoms of feet, or diffuse.

4 Sleep Issues
Diffuse 4-8 drops near bedside, or apply 1-2 drops to temples.

5 Focus Issues
Apply 1-2 drops to back of neck or temples.

6 Social Disorders
Inhale 1-2 drops from cupped hands, or rub onto back of neck.

Renewing Blend

place sticker _known name_ _____

Application

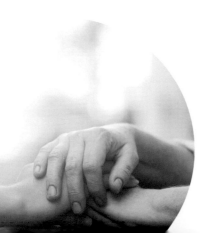 A T I

Main Ingredients
Spruce, Bergamot, Juniper Berry, Myrrh, Arborvitae, Citronella, Thyme, Nootka

Other Uses
Bitterness, Emotional Stagnation, Kidney Stones, Liver Issues, Muscle Pain, Sadness, Shame, Skin Infection

Top *Uses*

1 Anger, Resentment, Guilt
Apply 1-2 drops to pulse points, and inhale from cupped hands.

2 Attachment Issues
Apply 1-2 drops to pulse points, and diffuse.

3 Critical Thinking
Apply 1-2 drops to temples and back of neck, and diffuse.

4 Circulation
Apply 2-4 drops to bottoms of feet.

5 Insect Repellent
Apply with carrier oil over exposed skin.

6 Prostate Issues
Apply 1-2 drops over lower abdomen.

7 Irritability
Inhale 1-2 drops from cupped hands.

Oil Blends

Respiratory Blend

place sticker | *known name* _____

Application
A T I

Main Ingredients
Laurel, Eucalyptus, Peppermint, Melaleuca, Lemon, Cardamom, Ravintsara

Other Uses
Constricted Breathing, Emphysema, Exercise-Induced Asthma, Nasal Polyps, Respiratory Infections, Sinusitis, Tuberculosis

Safety
Can irritate sensitive skin. Use with caution during pregnancy.

Top *Uses*

1 Cough, Bronchitis, Pneumonia
Inhale 2-4 drops from cupped hands, and apply diluted over chest.

2 Asthma
Inhale 2-4 drops from cupped hands, and apply to lung reflex points.

3 Cold & Flu
Diffuse 5-10 drops, or apply with carrier oil over chest.

4 Allergies
Apply 1-2 drops over bridge of nose and sinuses, avoiding eyes.

5 Snoring
Apply 1-2 drops over throat and bridge of nose, avoiding eyes.

6 Closed off from Love
Rub a few drops over heart.

Restful Blend

place sticker *known name* _____

Application

A T I

Main Ingredients

Lavender, Sweet Marjoram, Chamomile, Ylang Ylang, Sandalwood, Cedarwood, Vetiver, Vanilla

Other Uses

Addictions, Hyperactivity, Insomnia, Lock Jaw, Mental Fatigue, Temporomandibular Joint Disorder (TMJ), Tension

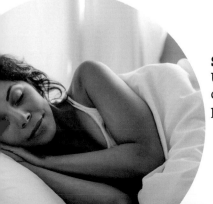

Safety
Use with caution during pregnancy.

Top *Uses*

1 Sleep Issues
Apply 1-2 drops to temples and bottoms of feet, and diffuse near bedside.

2 Stress & Anxiety
Apply 1-2 drops to pulse points, and inhale from cupped hands.

3 ADD & ADHD
Apply 1-2 drops to back of neck, and diffuse.

4 Itchy Skin
Apply 1-2 drops with carrier oil to affected areas.

5 Anger & Restlessness
Massage 1-2 drops into back of neck.

6 Hormone Balance & Mood Swings
Apply 1-2 drops to pulse points, or diffuse.

Skin Clearing Blend

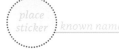

place sticker *known name* _____

Application

 ^A ^T ^I

Main Ingredients

Black Cumin, Ho Wood, Melaleuca, Geranium, Eucalyptus, Litsea

Top *Uses*

1 Acne & Blemishes
Apply directly to areas of concern.

2 Skin Impurities
Rub into skin before washing.

3 Oily Skin
Apply to areas of concern.

4 Eczema & Dermatitis
Apply with carrier oil to affected areas.

5 Bacterial Infection
Apply to affected areas.

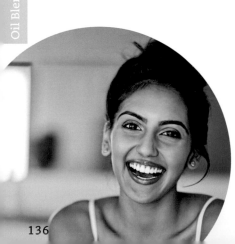

Safety
Possible skin irritation.

Soothing Blend

known name _____

Application

○ A ○ T ○ I

Main Ingredients
Wintergreen, Camphor, Peppermint, Blue Tansy, Helichrysum, Blue Chamomile

Other Uses
Back Pain, Bursitis, Frozen Shoulder, Growing Pains, Injured Joints, Tendinitis, Tennis Elbow, Workout (Pre and Post)

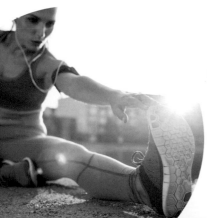

Safety
Can irritate sensitive skin. Use with caution during pregnancy.

Top _Uses_

1 Muscle Pain & Inflammation
Massage 2-4 drops with carrier oil or lotion into affected areas.

2 Joint Pain & Arthritis
Apply 1-2 drops to affected areas.

3 Lupus & Fibromyalgia
Apply 1-2 drops with carrier oil when experiencing flare-ups.

4 Whiplash
Apply 2-4 drops to affected areas.

5 Bruises
Gently apply 1-2 drops to bruising.

6 Headache
Apply 1-2 drops to temples and back of neck.

7 Bone Pain
Apply 2-4 drops directly over pain.

Tension Blend

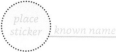
known name _____

Application

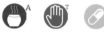

Main Ingredients
Wintergreen, Lavender, Peppermint, Frankincense, Cilantro, Marjoram, Chamomile, Rosemary

Other Uses
Alertness, Calming, Inflammation, Muscle Cramps, Swelling

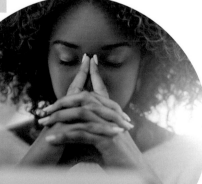

Safety
Can irritate sensitive skin. Use with caution during pregnancy.

Top *Uses*

1 Headache & Migraine
Massage into temples and forehead, avoiding eyes.

2 Muscle Tension
Massage into areas of concern.

3 Hot Flashes
Apply to back of neck.

4 Fevers
Apply to back of neck.

5 Bruises
Apply gently over bruises.

6 Hangover
Apply to temples and over stomach.

7 Arthritis
Massage into aching joints.

Oil Blends

Uplifting Blend

known name _____

Application

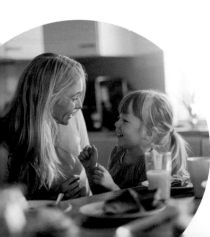

🍵 A 🖐 T 💊 I

Main Ingredients
Orange, Clove, Star Anise, Lemon Myrtle, Nutmeg, Ginger, Cinnamon, Zdravetz

Other Uses
Digestive Discomfort, Food Addiction, Jaw Pain, Lock Jaw, Low Energy

Safety
Can irritate sensitive skin. Use with caution during pregnancy.

Top *Uses*

1 Gloominess
Inhale 1-2 drops from cupped hands.

2 Self-Sabotage
Apply 1-2 drops over naval, and diffuse.

3 Low Energy
Apply 1-2 drops over adrenals on lower back, and diffuse.

4 Pessimism
Apply 1-2 drops to pulse points, and diffuse.

5 Detoxification
Apply 2-4 drops to bottoms of feet.

6 Emotional Disconnect
Apply 1-2 drops to temples or over heart.

7 Moodiness
Apply 1-2 drops to pulse points, or diffuse.

Oil Blends

139

Women's Blend

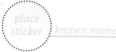

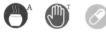 *known name*

Application

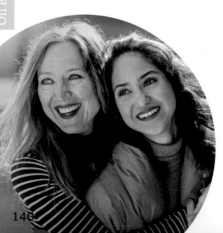

Main Ingredients
Bergamot, Ylang Ylang, Patchouli, Jasmine, Vanilla, Cinnamon, Labdanum, Vetiver, Cocoa, Rose

Other Uses
Loss of Vision, Skin Irritation

Oil Blends

Top *Uses*

1 Perfume
Apply 1-2 drops to pulse points.

2 Hormone Balance
Apply 1-2 drops to pulse points and back of neck.

3 Aphrodisiac
Apply 1-2 drops to neck and wrists.

4 Sedative & Calming
Inhale 1-2 drops from cupped hands.

5 Low Sex Drive
Apply 1-2 drops to pulse points.

6 Menopause
Apply 1-2 drops to pulse points.

Women's Monthly Blend

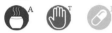

place sticker *known name* _____

Application

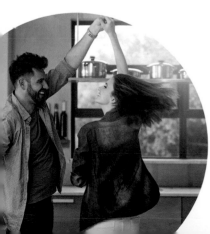

A   T   I

Main Ingredients

Clary Sage, Lavender, Bergamot, Chamomile, Cedarwood, Ylang Ylang, Geranium, Fennel, Carrot Seed, Palmarosa, Vitex

Other Uses

Aphrodisiac, Sedative, Sleep Issues

Safety

Avoid sun exposure for 12 hours after topical use.

Top *Uses*

1 PMS
Apply to wrists and over lower abdomen.

2 Cramping
Apply to lower abdomen.

3 Hormone Balance
Apply to wrists and over lower abdomen.

4 Hot Flashes
Apply to wrists and back of neck.

5 Mood Swings
Inhale from cupped hands, and apply to pulse points.

6 Self-Confidence
Inhale from cupped hands, and apply to pulse points.

7 Heavy Menstruation
Apply to lower abdomen.

Oil Blends

141

Section 6

Supplements
& Softgels

Vitality Supplement Set (trio)

known name _____

Components
- Cellular Vitality Complex
- Essential Oil + Omegas
- Food Nutrient Complex

Key Uses
- Vitality & Wellness
- Immune System Support
- Pain & Inflammation
- Sleep
- Mood, Depression, Anxiety
- Energy
- Hormone Balance
- Provides bio-available crucial nutrients to cells for building healthy organs, tissues, and body systems.

Supplements

Bone Nutrient

place sticker *known name* _____

Main Ingredients
Calcium (coral calcium), Vitamin C, Vitamin D-2, Biotin, Magnesium, Zinc, Copper, Manganese, Boron

Key Uses
- Promotes Bone Health
- Prevents age-related calcium loss
- Maintains bone mineralization
- Maximizes calcium utilization

Cellular Complex Softgel

place sticker *known name* _____

Main Ingredients
Frankincense, Orange, Lemongrass, Thyme, Summer Savory, Niaouli, Clove

Key Uses
- Aids in elimination of unhealthy cells
- Facilitates DNA repair
- Promotes healthy cellular function
- Useful for cancer, tumors, inflammation, infections, nervous system issues, immune system issues

Cellular Vitality Complex

place sticker *known name* _____

Main Ingredients
Boswellia Serrata, Scuttelaria Root, Milk Thistle, Pineapple Extract, Polygonum Capsudatum, Tumeric Root, Red Rasperry, Grape Seed, Marigold Flower, Tomato Fruit

Key Uses
- Protects body against free radicals
- Maintains proper cellular function
- Improves cellular vitality & energy
- Reduces inflammation

Children's Chewable

place sticker *known name* _____

Main Ingredients
Vitamins A, C, D, E, B1, B2, B3, B6, B12, B5, Folic Acid, Biotin, Calcium, Iron, Iodine, Magnesium, Zinc, Copper, Manganese, Superfood Blend, Cellular Vitality Blend

Key Uses
- Complete daily nutrient for children
- Food-derived nutrients
- Easy to ingest
- Pairs perfectly with other supplements

Supplements

145

Children's Omega-3

known name

Main Ingredients
Fish Oil (EPA, DHA), Vitamin D, Vitamin E, Vitamin C, Orange Essential Oil

Key Uses
- Provides benefits of fish oil without fishy taste
- Easy to take plain, or add to juice
- Supports brain, joint, and cardiovascular development

Children's Probiotic

known name

Main Ingredients
Lactobacillus Rhamnosus, Lactobacillus Salivarius, Lactobaccilus Plantarum LP01 & LP02, Bifidobacterium Breve, Bifidobacterium Lactis

Key Uses
- 5 billion live cells of 6 strains of flora
- Supports healthy digestive, neurological, immune, and brain function
- Shelf-stable unique delivery process

Daily Supplement (duo)

known name

Components
Food Nutrient Complex, Essential Oil + Omegas

Key Uses
- Provides complete daily nutrients derived from whole foods
- Complex omegas without standard preservatives, combined with essential oils
- Bioavailable nutrients to support body systems, organs, and cellular health

Detox Herbal Complex

known name

Main Ingredients
Psyllium Seed Husk, Barberry Leaf, Turkish Rhubarb, Kelp, Milk Thistle, Osha Root, Safflower, Acacia Gum, Burdoc, Root, Clove, Enzyme Assimilation Complex

Key Uses
- Whole-food Detox Herbal Complex
- Promotes healthy endocrine system
- Promotes toxin filtration
- Compliments Detoxification Blend

Detoxification Softgels

place sticker *known name*

Main Ingredients
Tangerine, Rosemary, Geranium, Juniper Berry, Cilantro

Key Uses
- Endocrine Support
- Promotes release of toxins
- Hormone Balance
- Antioxidant
- Stimulates adrenals
- Cleanses filtration organs

Digestion Comfort Tablets

place sticker *known name*

Main Ingredients
Cacium Carbonate, Ginger, Fennel, Coriander, Peppermint, Tarragon, Anise, Caraway

Key Uses
- Soothes GI discomfort
- Relieves heartburn and indigestion
- Relieves sour stomach
- Reduces belching and bloating

Digestive Enzymes

place sticker *known name*

Main Ingredients
Protcasc, Amylase, Lipase, Alpha Galactosidase, Cellulase, Maltase, Sucrase, Tummy Taming Blend, Enzyme Assimilation Blend

Key Uses
- Facilitates breakdown of food
- Increases nutrient absorption
- Promotes comfortable digestion
- Increases usability of nutrients
- Facilitates proper gut function

Digestive Blend Softgels

place sticker *known name*

Main Ingredients
Ginger, Peppermint, Tarragon, Fennel, Caraway, Coriander, Anise

Key Uses
- Soothes digestive discomfort
- Reduces gas and flatulence
- Reduces nausea
- Reduces diarrhea and constipation

Supplements

Energy & Stamina Complex

place sticker *known name*

Main Ingredients
Acetyl-L-Carnitine, Alpha-Lipolic Acid, Coenzyme Q10, Lychee Fruit, Green Tea Leaf, Quercetine Dihydrate, Cordyceps Mycelium, Ginseng, Ashwagandha

Key Uses
- Increases cellular energy
- Improves microcirculation
- Stimulates mitochondria
- Improves stamina

Essential Oil + Omegas

place sticker *known name*

Main Ingredients
Fish Oil (EPA DHA), Astaxanthin, Flaxseed Oil, Borage Seed Oil, Cranberry Seed Oil, Pomegranate Seed Oil, Vitamin D

Key Uses
- Promotes heart, brain, joint, eye, skin, and circulatory health
- Protects against lipid oxidation
- Molecularly filtered fish oil combined with internal dose of 9 essential oils

Food Nutrient Complex

place sticker *known name*

Main Ingredients
Vitamins A, C, D, E, K, B6, B12, Thiamin, Riboflavin, Niacin, Folate, Biotin, Pantothenic Acid, Calcium, Iron, Iodine, Magnesium, Zinc, Selenium, Copper, Manganese

Key Uses
- Whole-food comprehensive vitamin and mineral nutrient
- Provides bioavailable crucial nutrients to body systems, organs, and cells

Fruit & Veggie Drink Mix

place sticker *known name*

Main Ingredients
Kale, Dandelion, Collard Greens, Wheat Grass, Alfalfa, Barley Grass, Goji Berry, Mangosteen, Lemon & Ginger Oil

Key Uses
- Provides essential nutrients
- Supports Immune Health
- Supports Digestive Health
- Supports Weight Loss
- All natural ingredients

GI Cleansing Complex

place sticker *known name* _____

Main Ingredients
Caprylic Acid; Oregano, Melaleuca, Lemon, Lemongrass, and Thyme Oils

Key Uses
- Helps rid gut of parasites, Candida, and other harmful agents
- Supports healthy digestive environment
- Helps improve microbial balance

Phytoestrogen Complex

place sticker *known name* _____

Main Ingredients
Soy Extract (64% isoflavones, 50% Genistein), Flaxseed Extract (40% Lignan), Pomegranate Extract (40% Ellagic Acid)

Key Uses
- Promotes hormone balance by blocking estrogen binding to cells
- Manages harmful metabolite byproducts of hormone metabolism

Polyphenol Complex

place sticker *known name* _____

Main Ingredients
Frankincense Extract, Turmeric, Ginger, Green Tea Extract, Pomegranate Extract, Grape Seed Extract, Resveratrol

Key Uses
- Reduces inflammation and pain
- Provides relief to tension headaches, as well as back, neck, and shoulder pain
- Antioxidant support
- Internal compliment to Soothing Blend

Probiotic Complex

place sticker *known name* _____

Main Ingredients
L. acidophilus, B. lactis, L. salivarius, L. casei, B. longum, B. bifidum

Key Uses
- 6 billion CFUs
- Supports digestive & immune systems
- Unique double-encapsulated delivery
- Shelf stable with prebiotics to sustain probiotics
- Helps digestion of food nutrients

Supplements

Protective Softgels +

place sticker *known name* _____

Main Ingredients
Clove, Wild Orange, Black Pepper, Cinnamon, Eucalyptus, Oregano, Rosemary, Melissa

Key Uses
· Supercharged Protective Blend
· Combats viral and bacterial infections
· Supports immune system

Restful Complex

place sticker *known name* _____

Main Ingredients
Lavender, L-theanine, Lemonbalm, Passion Flower, Chamomile

Key Uses
· Promotes falling asleep faster
· Supports more meaningful sleep
· Promotes waking up feeling refreshed

Seasonal Blend Softgels

place sticker *known name* _____

Main Ingredients
Lemon, Lavender, & Peppermint Essential Oils

Key Uses
· Reduces hysthamine response
· Opens airways
· Relieves itchiness
· Eases sinus congestion
· Useful for seasonal and pet allergies

Trim Shake

place sticker *known name* _____

Main Ingredients
Whey & Egg White Protein, Fiber Blend, Stevia, Annatto, Ashwagandha, Potato Protein, Trim Complex

Key Uses
· Meal replacement shake
· Reduces cortisol levels to reduce fat retention
· Manages appetite and cravings
· Healthy protein-carb-fat ratio

Section 7

Protocols

Acne (bacteria)

Description
Combats bacterial overgrowth that becomes trapped in pores.

Suggested Duration
Ongoing

Skin Clearing Blend
Apply a small amount evenly over clean skin after showering daily.

Melaleuca
Apply a dab to blemishes.

Frankincense
Apply a dab to healing blemishes to prevent scarring.

Additional Support
• Anti-Aging Blend

Acne (hormones)

Description
Balances hormone production and maintenance throughout the body, including the gut.

Suggested Duration
Until desired appearance is achieved, then as needed

Vitality Supplement Trio
Take 2 of each supplement twice daily.

Phytoestrogen Complex
Take 1 capsule with each dose of Vitality Supplements (for men and women).

Clary Sage
Rub 1 drop on pulse points before bed.

Skin Clearing Blend
Apply a small amount to blemishes daily as needed.

Acne (toxicity)

Description
Alleviates toxicity overload by detoxing organs and skin.

Suggested Duration
3-5 weeks

Detoxification Softgels
Take 1 softgel with each meal.

Detox Herbal Complex
Take 1 capsule with breakfast and dinner.

Cellular Complex Softgels
Take 1 softgel with each meal.

Skin Clearing Blend
Apply small amount to blemishes daily as needed.

Additional Support
A 30-day full detox is highly recommended, including eliminating inflammatory foods from diet.

ADD/ADHD

Description
Increases focus and concentration, supports healthy hormones and brain chemistry.

Suggested Duration
Ongoing

Vitality Supplement Trio
Take 2 of each bottle 2x/day.

Focus Blend
Carry in your pocket, and roll a small amount on back of neck as needed for focus.

Grounding Blend
Apply 2 drops to bottoms of feet each morning.

Probiotic Complex
Take 1 with each meal.

Additional Support
- Restful Blend
- Restful Complex
- Wild Orange

Adrenal Fatigue

Description
Supports healthy adrenal function.

Suggested Duration
4-8 weeks

Lemon (8 drops), Basil (3), Rosemary (3), Frankincense (3)
Combine in roller bottle. Fill the rest with carrier oil. Massage into neck and kidneys daily as often as needed.

Rosemary & Peppermint
Breathe a drop of each from cupped hands, or diffuse for energy as needed.

Vitality Supplement Trio
Take 2 of each bottle 2x/day.

Energy & Stamina Complex
Take 2 capsules 2x/day.

Additional Support
- Invigorating Blend
- Detoxification Blend

AIDS/HIV

Description
Provides emotional support, promotes a properly functioning immune system.

Suggested Duration
6 months, then as needed

Joyful Blend
Carry with you, and inhale from hands for mood boost throughout the day.

Cellular Complex Blend
Rub 3-5 drops onto spine nightly.

Cellular Complex Softgels
Take 1 softgel 3x/day.

Vitality Supplement Trio
Take 2 of each bottle 2x/day.

Protective Blend
Rub 2 drops on bottoms of feet in the morning.

Protocols

Allergies (food)

Description
Lowers histamine response triggered by food allergies, and creates calm in the gut.

Suggested Duration
4 weeks to begin, then as needed

Lavender
Put 1 drop under tongue. Drink water after 30 seconds.

Probiotic Complex
Take 1 capsule 3x/day.

Polyphenol Complex
Take 1 capsule 3x/day.

Digestive Enzyme Complex
Take 1 with each meal.

Additional Support
· Do a 14-day bone broth cleanse
· Detox Herbal Complex
· Detoxification Blend

Allergies (pet/seasonal)

Description
Reduces histamine response and boosts immune response.

Suggested Duration
4-8 weeks to begin, then as needed

Lemon, Lavender, Peppermint
Put 1 drop each under tongue. Drink water after 30 seconds.

Respiratory Blend
Inhale from cupped hands when experiencing attack.

Probiotic Complex
Take 1 capsule 3x/day.

Protective Blend
Gargle 2 drops with water nightly, then swallow.

Additional Support
· Seasonal Blend Softgels
· White Fir
· Vitality Supplement Trio

Allergies (skin)

Description
Calms irritation due to skin contact with allergens.

Suggested Duration
As needed

Lavender, Helichrysum, Frankincense, Lemon
Combine 10 drops of each in a roller bottle. Fill the rest with carrier oil. Roll onto affected area often.

Lavender
Put a drop under tongue . Drink water after 30 seconds.

Probiotic Complex
Take 1 capsule 3x/day.

Additional Support
· Detox Herbal Complex
· Detoxification Blend

Alzheimer's

Description
Supports healthy mental activity, boosts alertness.

Suggested Duration
Ongoing

Vitality Supplement Trio
Take 2 of each bottle 2x/day.

Cellular Complex Blend
Rub 3-5 drops along spine or bottoms of feet daily.

Cellular Complex Softgels
Take 1 softgel 3x/day.

Peppermint & Rosemary
Diffuse daily to increase alertness & memory.

Additional Support
- Cilantro
- Frankincense
- Extra Omega-3's
- Grounding Blend

Anxiety

Description
Reduces stress levels, promotes sense of calm, security, and focus.

Suggested Duration
3-6 months, then as needed

Grounding Blend
Apply 2 drops to bottoms of feet in mornings. Rub a drop behind ears when anxious.

Frankincense
Put a drop under tongue. Drink water after 30 seconds.

Reassuring Blend
Apply to pulse points and temples as needed.

Vitality Supplement Trio
Take 2 of each bottle 2x/day.

Additional Support
- Patchouli
- Lavender
- Wild Orange

Arthritis

Description
Reduces inflammation in joints, supports joint function.

Suggested Duration
8 weeks to start, then as needed

Soothing Blend
Apply in lotion and massage into joints often as needed.

Polyphenol Complex
Take 1 capsule 2x/day.

Frankincense
Massage 2-4 drops into joints daily.

Lemongrass
Massage 1 drop diluted into joints after Soothing Blend or Frankincense.

Additional Support
- Massage Blend
- Wintergreen
- Peppermint

Asthma

Description
Promotes open airways and easy breathing.

Suggested Duration
As needed

Respiratory Blend
Inhale 2 drops from cupped hands during attack.

Lavender
Massage a drop behind ears to promote calm.

Cardamom
Gargle a drop for 30 seconds, then swallow as needed.

Additional Support
• Rosemary
• Siberian Fir
• Eucalyptus

Autism

Description
Promotes high-functioning mental activity, reduces heavy metal toxicity.

Suggested Duration
12 months

Cellular Complex Blend
Massage 5 drops into spine nightly.

Frankincense & Cilantro
Massage 2 drops each into bottoms of feet 2x/day.

Probiotic Complex
Take 1 capsule 3x/day (or use Children's Probiotic)

Essential Oil + Omega 3
Take 2 softgels 3x/day (or use Children's Omega 3)

Peppermint & Rosemary
Diffuse daily to stimulate healthy mental activity.

Back, Neck, Shoulder Pain

Description
Reduces pain and inflammation, restores mobility.

Suggested Duration
4 weeks, then as needed

Soothing Blend
Massage in lotion into affected areas often as needed.

Polyphenol Complex
Take 1 capsule 3x/day.

Vitality Supplement Trio
Take 2 of each bottle 2x/day.

Additional Support
• Yoga/stretching
• Massage Blend
• Marjoram
• Black Pepper

Bathroom Spray

Neutralizes bathroom odors without chemicals.

Hopefully at least once a day

Lemongrass, Lime, Grapefruit
Add 10 drops each to glass spray bottle. Fill with water. Add a bit of rubbing alcohol/vodka to eliminate the need to shake before use.

· Cleansing Blend
· Invigorating Blend
· Juniper Berry
· Melaleuca

Blood Pressure

Helps lower high blood pressure, promotes circulation.

4-8 weeks, then as needed

Cypress, Ylang Ylang, Marjoram
Rub a drop of each onto bottoms of feet every morning.

Frankincense, Ylang Ylang, Marjoram, Lemon
Take 1-2 drops each in capsule daily.

Vitality Supplement Trio
Take 2 of each bottle 2x/day.

· Reduce sodium intake
· Daily exercise
· Petitgrain
· Roman Chamomile

Bronchitis/ Pneumonia

Reduces coughing, boosts immune system, combats respiratory infection.

5-10 days

Lime, Rosemary, Siberian Fir
Rub 2 drops each onto chest, upper back, and bottoms of feet several times a day.

Cardamom
Gargle 2 drops with water, then swallow.

Respiratory Blend & Frankincense
Diffuse 3-5 drops each, and sit/sleep by the diffuser.

· Vitality Supplement Trio
· Thyme
· Eucalyptus

Cancer

Description
Promotes healthy cellular apoptosis and cellular function.

Suggested Duration
6-12 months

Cellular Complex Softgel
Take 1 softgel 3x/day.

Frankincense
Rub 3-5 drops as close to the affected area as possible 3x/day.

Sandalwood & Lavender
Diffuse daily.

Vitality Supplement Trio
Take 2 of each bottle 2x/day.

Additional Support
• Eat an alkaline diet
• Helichrysum
• Geranium

Candida

Description
Combats fungus overgrowth in gut, restores healthy flora.

Suggested Duration
4 weeks

GI Cleansing Complex
Take 1 softgel 3x/day with meals for 10 days (begin with only 1 a day, and work your way up).

Detoxification Softgels
Take 1 softgel 3x/day for 30 days.

Lemon
Drink 1-3 drops in water 3x/day.

Probiotic Complex
Take 1 capsule 3x/day after 10 days of GI Cleansing.

Additional Support
• Eliminate sugar & grains
• Melaleuca
• Thyme

Canker Sores

Description
Provides virus & bacteria support, reduces pain.

Suggested Duration
As needed

Frankincense, Melaleuca
Apply a drop of each diluted to the outside of cheek, over canker sore.

Melissa, Melaleuca
Use a drop of each heavily diluted directly onto canker sore.

Additional Support
• Protective Blend
• Clove
• Black Pepper

Carpet Deodorizer

Eliminates carpet odors from food and pets.

As needed

Cleansing Blend, Lemon, Lime, Melaleuca
Combine 5 drops each with 1 cup baking soda. Rub evenly throughout carpet, and let sit for 12-24 hours before vacuuming.

Additional Support
- Grapefruit
- Bergamot
- Douglas Fir

Celiac's

Description
Promotes nutrient absorption, calms digestive system.

Suggested Duration
Ongoing

Digestive Enzymes
Take 2-3 capsules with meals.

Digestive Blend
Rub on outside of stomach at onset of pain.

Metabolic Blend Softgels
Take 1-2 softgels 2-3x/day.

Additional Support:
- Cinnamon
- Grapefruit
- Frankincense

Cholesterol

Description
Helps return high cholesterol back to normal levels.

Suggested Duration
4-6 weeks

Marjoram & Lemongrass
Take 2 drops each in capsule daily.

Cypress & Grounding Blend
Massage 2 drops each into bottoms of feet each morning.

Additional Support
- Metabolic Blend
- Lemon
- Clary Sage
- Helichrysum

Cold Sores

Combats viral infection, and promotes skin healing and pain relief.

As needed

Melaleuca & Melissa
Apply a drop of each diluted several times a day.

Frankincense or Helichrysum
Apply a drop diluted between the Melaleuca & Melissa.

- Arborvitae
- Black Pepper
- Protective Blend

Colds

Provides antiviral and respiratory support.

5-10 days

Protective Blend Softgels
Take 1-2 softgels 3x/day.

Protective Blend, Black Pepper, Melaleuca
Rub 1-2 drops each on bottoms of feet 3x/day.

Respiratory Blend
Rub onto chest and diffuse as needed.

Vitality Supplement Trio
Take 2 of each bottle 2x/day.

- Rosemary
- Cardamom
- Lime
- Energy & Stamina Complex

Cough

Calms coughing and promotes restful breathing.

As needed

Peppermint, Rosemary, & Lime
Rub 2 drops of each onto chest and bottoms of feet.

Cardamom
Gargle 2 drops with water, then swallow.

Respiratory Blend
Diffuse, and sit/sleep by diffuser.

- Vitality Supplement Trio
- Eucalyptus

Crohn's

Description
Reduces inflammation and swelling in the bowels.

Suggested Duration
6 months

GI Cleansing Complex
Take 1 softgel 1-2x/day for 2 weeks.

Peppermint, Basil, Frankincense
Take 1-2 drops each in capsule daily for 2 weeks after GI Cleansing Complex.

Probiotic Complex
Take 1 capsule w/each meal.

Digestive Blend
Take as softgel or in water often as needed.

Additional Support
• Vitality Supplement Trio
• Ginger
• Marjoram

Deodorant (body)

Description
Helps manage bacteria and odor-causing toxicity.

Suggested Duration
4 weeks, then as needed

Cilantro
Take 2 drops in a capsule daily.

Detoxification Softgels
Take 1 softgel 2x/day.

Cleansing Blend
Use diluted with carrier oil under arms after showering.

Additional Support
• Joyful Blend
• Melaleuca
• Arborvitae
• Petitgrain

Depression

Description
Improves brain chemistry, supports healthy hormone production.

Suggested Duration
3-6 months, then as needed

Vitality Supplement Trio
Take 2 of each bottle 2x/day.

Essential Oil + Omegas
Take an extra dose of omegas daily.

Probiotic Complex
Take 1 capsule w/each meal.

Joyful Blend
Carry with you, and inhale from cupped hands often as needed for mood support.

Frankincense or Melissa
Put a drop under the tongue 1-3x/day.

Additional Support
• Encouraging Blend

Detox (full body)

Description
Helps the body eliminate toxicity and free up filtering organs.

Suggested Duration
4 weeks

GI Cleansing Complex
Take 1 softgel w/each meal for 10 days (start with 1 a day, and work up to 3).

Detoxification Softgels
Take 1 softgel w/each meal.

Detox Herbal Complex
Take 1 capsule 2x/day.

Lemon
Drink 1-3 drops with water 3x/day.

Probiotic Complex
Take 1 capsule w/each meal during last 10 days.

Vitality Supplement Trio
Take 2 of each bottle 2x/day.

Diabetes (type 1)

Description
Stimulates cellular maintenance, helps balance blood sugar.

Suggested Duration
3-6 months, then as needed

Vitality Supplement Trio
Take 2 of each bottle 2x/day.

Rosemary, Cypress, Cassia
Take 1 drop each in capsule daily. Also rub diluted onto pancreas reflex points.

Geranium & Rosemary
Add 3 drops of each to a hot bath.

Additional Support
• Cellular Complex Blend
• Coriander
• Juniper Berry
• Bergamot

Diabetes (type 2)

Description
Helps balance blood sugar, supports pancreas.

Suggested Duration
3-6 months, then as needed

Coriander, Cinnamon, Juniper Berry
Take 1-2 drops each in capsule daily.

Cellular Vitality Complex
Take 2 of each bottle 2x/day.

Detoxification Blend
Rub 2 drops onto pancreas reflex point or over pancreas daily.

Additional Support
• Cassia
• Metabolic Blend

Digestive Issues

Description
Relieves inflammation, gas, and discomfort in digestive system.

Suggested Duration
2-4 weeks, then as needed

Digestive Blend
Drink 1-2 drops with water, or rub over stomach to ease discomfort.

Digestive Enzymes
Take 1 capsule w/each meal.

Probiotic Complex
Take 1 capsule w/each meal.

Frankincense & Cardamom
Rub a drop of each onto stomach reflex points in the morning.

Additional Support
- Ginger
- Fennel
- Peppermint

Eczema/Dermatitis

Description
Relieves itchiness, promotes skin repair.

Suggested Duration
2-4 weeks

Roller Bottle
Combine 10 drops of Frankincense, Lavender, Melaleuca, Helichrysum, 3 drops Black Pepper, and fill the rest with carrier oil. Use several times a day.

Detox Herbal Complex
Take 1 capsule 2x/day.

Probiotic Complex
Take 1 capsule w/each meal.

Additional Support
- Anti-Aging Blend
- Cedarwood
- Copaiba

Fatigue (low energy)

Description
Supports adrenals, microcirculation, and alertness.

Suggested Duration
4 weeks, then as needed

Vitality Supplement Trio
Take 2 of each bottle 2x/day.

Energy & Stamina Complex
Take 2 capsules 2x/day.

Peppermint & Rosemary
Apply 2 drops to bottoms of feet daily. Inhale from cupped hands as needed.

Lemon or Grapefruit
Use 1-3 drops in water 3x/day.

Additional Support:
- Invigorating Blend
- Uplifting Blend
- Neroli
- Basil

Protocols

Fibromyalgia

Description
Decreases inflammation, promotes healthy cellular function.

Suggested Duration
2-6 months

Full Body Detox
Follow instructions for Detox (full body).

Vitality Supplement Trio
Take 2 of each bottle 2x/day.

Polyphenol Complex
Take 1 capsule 3x/day.

Soothing Blend
Massage into inflamed areas.

Cellular Complex Softgels
Take 1 softgel 3x/day.

Additional Support
• Probiotic Complex
• Detoxification Blend
• Restful Blend
• Wild Orange

Flu Bomb

Description
Combats viruses, boosts immune system, supports respiratory system.

Suggested Duration
5-10 days

Oregano, Melaleuca, Protective Blend, Lemon
Take 1-2 drops of each in a capsule 3x/day.

Digestive Blend
Drink 1-3 drops in water, or rub over stomach to ease nausea & vomiting.

Respiratory Blend
Diffuse 8-10 drops. Sit/sleep near the diffuser.

Additional Support
• Black Pepper
• Melissa
• Cardamom
• Protective Blend+ Softgels
• GI Cleansing Complex

Heartburn

Description
Balances stomach acid, eases pain of indigestion.

Suggested Duration
As needed

Digestive Blend
Drink 1-2 drops in water.

Digestive Enzymes
Take 1-3 capsules with each meal.

Cardamom
Rub 1-2 drops over stomach.

Additional Support
• Ginger
• Fennel
• Coriander

Immune Boost

Provides bacteria and virus-fighting agents, boosts immune system.

4 weeks

Protective Blend, Black Pepper, Melaleuca
Rub a drop of each on bottoms of feet daily.

Probiotic Complex
Take 1 capsule w/each meal.

Vitality Supplement Trio
Take 2 of each bottle 2x/day.

• Frankincense
• Melissa
• Thyme

Infertility

Supports the reproductive system and proper hormone production.

2-6 months

Full Body Detox
Follow instructions for Detox (full body).

Vitality Supplement Trio
Take 2 of each bottle 2x/day.

Clary Sage
Apply to reproductive reflex points 2x/day.

• Oil Touch Technique (receive weekly)
• Detoxification Blend

Irritable Bowels (IBS)

Calms chronic digestive irritation and diarrhea.

2-4 weeks

Digestive Blend
Drink 1-2 drops with water after eating.

Digestive Enzymes
Take 1-3 capsules with meals.

Frankincense & Ginger
Massage a drop of each into stomach/bowels reflex points.

Grounding Blend
Rub a drop behind ears to manage stress as needed.

• Cardamom
• Coriander

Libido (sex drive)

Description
Inspires uninhibited sex drive.

Suggested Duration
2 weeks, then as needed

Inspiring Blend
Use a few drops diluted in massage, and diffuse to inspire intimacy.

Ylang Ylang
Rub 1-2 drops on pulse points.

Clary Sage
Take 1-2 drops in capsule daily.

Additional Support
• Vitality Supplement Trio
• Energy & Stamina Complex

Lupus

Description
Reduces inflammation, supports cellular function.

Suggested Duration
6-12 months

Soothing Blend
Massage into inflamed areas often as needed.

Vitality Supplement Trio
Take 2 of each bottle 2x/day.

Polyphenol Complex
Take 1 capsule 3x/day.

Cellular Complex
Rub 5 drops along spine every night.

Additional Support
• Frankincense
• Probiotic Complex
• Grounding Blend
• Joyful Blend

Lyme Disease

Description
Provides strong antibacterial support, reduces inflammation.

Suggested Duration
2 week intervals with 1 week rest in between as needed

Cinnamon, Oregano, Thyme, Clove
Take 2 drops each in a capsule 1-2x/day.

Frankincense, Black Pepper
Massage 1-2 drops over lymph nodes daily.

Vitality Supplement Trio
Take 2 of each bottle 2x/day.

Additional Support
• Melissa
• Protective Blend
• Energy & Stamina Complex

Menopause

Aids in hormone and mood balance, calms hot flashes.

4 months, then as needed

Women's Monthly Blend
Rub onto pulse points twice daily (avoid sun exposure for 12 hours after application).

Phytoestrogen Complex
Take 1 capsule 3x/day.

Peppermint
Apply a drop to back of neck to ease hot flashes.

• Vitality Supplement Trio
• Ylang Ylang
• Geranium

Menstruation

Balances mood and hormones during menstruation.

2 weeks as needed

Women's Monthly Blend
Rub onto pulse points and over ovaries (avoid sun exposure for 12 hours after application).

Balance
Rub behind ears to balance mood.

Phytoestrogen
Take 1 capsule 3x/day.

• Clary Sage
• Restful Blend
• Tension Blend

Mononucleosis

Provides antiviral support.

2-4 weeks

Thyme, Oregano, Protective Blend
Take 1-2 drops each in a capsule 3x/day.

Frankincense, Black Pepper
Rub 2 drops each to bottoms of feet.

Energy & Stamina Complex
Take 1-2 capsules twice daily.

• Vitality Supplement Trio
• Melissa
• Cassia

Muscle Aches

Description
Reduces inflammation, spasms, and pain in muscles.

Suggested Duration
2 weeks, then as needed

Massage Blend
Massage 2-4 drops into aching muscles 3x/day.

Polyphenol Complex
Take 1 capsule 3x/day.

Frankincense, Lemon
Take 1-2 drops each in capsule 2x/day.

Additional Support
- Soothing Blend
- Cypress
- Douglas Fir
- Black Pepper

Pregnancy (postnatal)

Description
Promotes pain relief, tissue healing, and emotional support after giving birth.

Suggested Duration
4-8 weeks

Helichrysum, Frankincense, Lavender
Apply 2 drops each diluted to areas with tearing 3x/day.

Ylang Ylang
Diffuse for mood balancing.

Phytoestrogen
Take 1 capsule 3x/day.

Helichrysum, Myrrh, Lavender
Massage 2 drops each diluted into stretch mark areas.

Additional Support
- Geranium
- Vitality Supplement Trio

Pregnancy (prenatal)

Description
Relieves pregnancy sickness, provides vital nutrients, and provides emotional support.

Suggested Duration
9 months

Digestive Blend
Drink 2 drops or rub 2 drops over stomach to ease nausea.

Digestive Enzymes
Take 1-3 w/each meal.

Vitality Supplement Trio
Take 2 of each bottle 2x/day.

Bone Nutrient Complex
Take 1 capsule 3x/day.

Joyful Blend
Diffuse or wear daily.

Additional Support
- Ginger
- Grounding Blend
- Metabolic Blend
- Rose

Psoriasis

Description
Relieves itchy, swollen skin, and promotes proper immune system function.

Suggested Duration
4-8 weeks

Helichrysum, Frankincense, Melaleuca, Lavender
Combine 10 drops each with carrier oil in roller bottle. Apply 3x/day.

Probiotic Complex
Take 1 capsule 3x/day.

Digestive Enzymes
Take 1-3 w/each meal.

Cellular Complex Blend
Take 1-2 softgels 3x/day.

Additional Support
• Copaiba
• Anti-Aging Blend
• Cedarwood

Shingles

Description
Provides antiviral support and viral detox.

Suggested Duration
4 weeks, then as needed

Melaleuca, Melissa, Black Pepper
Take 1-2 drops in capsule 3x/day.

Frankincense, Lavender
Apply 2 drops each diluted to affected areas.

Vitality Supplement Trio
Take 2 of each bottle 2x/day.

Detoxification Blend
Rub 2 drops on bottoms of feet before showering.

Additional Support
• Lime
• Protective Blend
• Cedarwood

Sinus Bomb

Description
Helps fight sinus infection.

Suggested Duration
5-10 days

Myrrh, Oregano, Frankincense, Lemon
Combine 10 drops each (3 drops of Oregano) with carrier oil in roller bottle. Apply carefully over cheek bones and brow, avoiding eyes, 3-5x/day.

Oregano, Thyme
Take 1-2 drops each in capsule 3x/day.

Additional Support
• Protective Blend
• Respiratory Blend
• Eucalyptus

Sleep Apnea

Description
Promotes open airways and more meaningful sleep.

Suggested Duration
Ongoing

Respiratory Blend
Diffuse 5-10 drops next to bedside at night. Also apply to sinus reflex points.

Protective Blend
Gargle 2 drops with water for 30 seconds, then swallow.

Restful Complex
Take 2 softgels 30 minutes before bed.

Additional Support
- Peppermint
- Rosemary
- Wintergreen

Sleep/Insomnia

Description
Supports falling and staying asleep, and to wake feeling more rested.

Suggested Duration
4 weeks, then as needed

Restful Blend
Diffuse 5-10 drops next to bedside at night. Also apply to temples and bottoms of feet before bed.

Restful Complex
Take 2 softgels 30 minutes before bed.

Wild Orange
Put a drop under tongue before bed.

Additional Support
- Melissa
- Vetiver
- Cedarwood
- Roman Chamomile
- Vitality Supplement Trio

Smoking

Description
Helps curb cravings and smoking addiction, aids in detox.

Suggested Duration
6-12 weeks

Grapefruit
Drink 1-3 drops in water throughout the day.

Protective Blend
Swish 2 drops with water when cravings arise, especially after eating.

Black Pepper
Apply 1 drop to big toes 2x/day. Also inhale or diffuse throughout the day.

Detoxification Softgels
Take 1 softgel 3x/day.

Additional Support
- Clove
- Detox Herbal Complex

Snoring

Description
Promotes open airways during sleep.

Suggested Duration
Ongoing

Respiratory Blend
Diffuse 5-10 drops near bedside at night. Also apply to chest, throat, and lung reflex points.

Protective Blend
Gargle 2 drops with water for 30 seconds, then swallow.

Lemon
Drink 1-3 drops in water before bed.

Additional Support
• Eucalyptus
• Rosemary
• Peppermint

Sore Throat

Description
Relieves pain and soreness in throat, provides antiviral and antibacterial support.

Suggested Duration
5-10 days

Lemon 10, Protective Blend 8, Helichrysum 2
Combine in small glass spray bottle with carrier oil. Apply as needed.

Lavender, Arborvitae
Massage 1-2 drops with carrier oil to outside of throat.

Additional Support
• Melissa
• Black Pepper
• Petitgrain

Stress-Away

Description
Reduces excess levels of cortisol, balances emotions.

Suggested Duration
4 weeks, then as needed

Grounding Blend
Apply 1-2 drops to back of ears, temples, and wrists often as needed.

Frankincense
Diffuse daily.

Lavender
Take 1-2 drops in capsule 2x/day.

Additional Support
• Reassuring Blend
• Ylang Ylang
• Spikenard
• Invigorating Blend

Sunburn

Description
Relieves discomfort from sunburn, promotes healing.

Suggested Duration
3-7 days

Lavender, Helichrysum
Apply 2-4 drops with carrier oil or aloe to sunburnt skin 3-5x/day.

Peppermint
Add 5 drops to small glass spray bottle with water. Spritz to cool skin.

Additional Support
- Cedarwood
- Copaiba
- Roman Chamomile

Thrush

Description
Provides anti-fungal support, eases oral discomfort.

Suggested Duration
1-3 weeks

Lemon, Melaleuca, Children's Omega-3
Combine 2 drops of each essential oil with 1 Tbs of omegas. Apply with clean finger to child's gums and tongue 2-3x/day.

Melaleuca & Lavender
Massage a drop into bottoms of child's feet 1x/day.

Additional Support
- Geranium
- Helichrysum

Thyroid: Hyper (Grave's)

Description
Calms an overactive thyroid, balances thyroid hormones.

Suggested Duration
4-6 months

Myrrh, Frankincense, Rosemary
Combine 10 drops each in roller bottle, fill remaining with carrier oil. Apply over thyroid 3x/day.

Cellular Complex Softgels
Take 1 softgel 3x/day

Probiotic Complex
Take 1 capsule w/each meal.

Additional Support
- Lemongrass

Thyroid: Hypo (Hashimoto's)

Description
Stimulates thyroid in order to produce proper hormones.

Suggested Duration
4-6 months

Clove, Myrrh, Lemongrass, Peppermint
Combine 10 drops each in roller bottle, fill remaining with carrier oil. Apply over thyroid 3-5x/day. Also take a drop of each in capsule 3x/day for first week.

Cellular Complex Blend
Apply a drop to thyroid reflex point daily.

Energy & Stamina Complex
Take 2 capsules 2x/day.

Additional Support
· Bergamot
· Spearmint
· Vitality Supplement Trio

Weight loss

Description
Stimulates metabolism, curbs appetite, aids in detox.

Suggested Duration
4-12 weeks

Metabolic Blend Softgels
Take 1-3 softgels 3x/day.

Grapefruit & Peppermint
Drink 1-3 drops in water throughout the day to curb cravings.

Energy & Stamina Complex
Take 2 capsules 2x/day.

Detoxification Softgels
Take 1 softgel 3x/day.

Additional Support
· Detox Herbal Complex
· Digestive Enzymes
· Lemon

Workout

Description
Provides pre- and post-workout support, increases energy, supports muscle tone.

Suggested Duration
Ongoing

Massage Blend
Apply 1-3 drops to muscles to stimulate circulation before workout.

Respiratory Blend
Apply 2-4 drops to chest to open airways.

Energy & Stamina Complex
Take 2 capsules before workout, and 2 with dinner.

Soothing Blend
Apply in lotion to muscles and joints after workout. Add Marjoram if injured.

Additional Support
· Lemongrass
· Vitality Supplement Trio

Protocols

Bibliography

Aromatic Science. AromaticScience, LLC. Web. July, 2017. <www.aromaticscience.com>

Enlighten Alternative Healing. Emotions and Essential Oils: A Modern Resource for Healing: Emotional Reference Guide. 3rd ed., Enlighten Alternative Healing, 2016.

Harding, Jennie: The Essential Oils Handbook. Duncan Baird Publishers Ltd, 2008.

Lawless, Julia: The Encyclopedia of Essential Oils: The Complete Guide to the Use of Aromatic Oils In Aromatherapy, Herbalism, Health, and Well Being. Conari Press, 2013.

Schiller, Carol & Schiller, David: The Aromatherapy Encyclopedia: A Concise Guide to Over 395 Plant Oils. Basic Health Publications Inc, 2008.

Schnaubelt, Kurt. The Healing Intelligence of Essential Oils: the Science of Advanced Aromatherapy. Healing Arts Press, 2011.

Tisserand, Robert, et al. Essential Oil Safety: A Guide for Health Care Professionals. 2nd ed., Churchill Livingstone/Elsevier, 2014.

Worwood, Valerie Ann. The Complete Book of Essential Oils and Aromatherapy, Revised and Expanded: Over 800 Natural, Nontoxic, and Fragrant Recipes to Create Health, Beauty, And Safe Home and Work Environments. New World Library, 2016.

Section 8

Protocols
for sharing

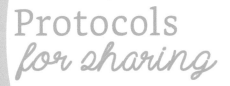

ADD/ADHD

Description
Increases focus and concentration, supports healthy hormones and brain chemistry.

Suggested Duration
Ongoing

Vitality Supplement Trio
Take 2 of each bottle 2x/day.

Focus Blend
Carry in your pocket, and roll a small amount on back of neck as needed for focus.

Grounding Blend
Apply 2 drops to bottoms of feet each morning.

Probiotic Complex
Take 1 with each meal.

ADD/ADHD

Description
Increases focus and concentration, supports healthy hormones and brain chemistry.

Suggested Duration
Ongoing

Vitality Supplement Trio
Take 2 of each bottle 2x/day.

Focus Blend
Carry in your pocket, and roll a small amount on back of neck as needed for focus.

Grounding Blend
Apply 2 drops to bottoms of feet each morning.

Probiotic Complex
Take 1 with each meal.

"Health is the greatest gift, content-
ment is the greatest wealth, faithful-
ness the best relationship."

-Buddha

This protocol is
brought to you by the book
Essential Oil Magic

"A calm mind brings inner strength
and self-confidence."

-Dalai Lama

This protocol is
brought to you by the book
Essential Oil Magic

Allergies

Description
Reduces histamine response, boosts immune response.

Suggested Duration
4-8 weeks to begin, then as needed

Lemon, Lavender, Peppermint
Put 1 drop each under tongue. Drink water after 30 seconds.

Respiratory Blend
Inhale from cupped hands when experiencing attack.

Probiotic Complex
Take 1 capsule 3x/day.

Protective Blend
Gargle 2 drops with
water nightly,
then swallow.

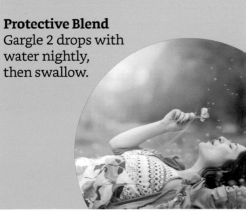

"In three words I can sum up everything I've learned about life: It goes on."

-Robert Frost

This protocol is
brought to you by the book
Essential Oil Magic

"As for butter versus margarine, I trust cows more than chemists."

-Joan Gussow

This protocol is
brought to you by the book
Essential Oil Magic

Anxiety & Stress

Description
Reduces stress levels, promotes sense of calm, security, and focus.

Suggested Duration
3-6 months, then as needed

Grounding Blend
Apply 2 drops to bottoms of feet in mornings. Rub a drop behind ears when anxious.

Frankincense
Put a drop under tongue. Drink water after 30 seconds.

Reassuring Blend
Apply to pulse points and temples as needed.

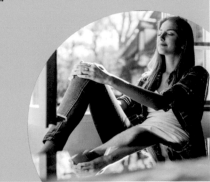

Anxiety & Stress

Description
Reduces stress levels, promotes sense of calm, security, and focus.

Suggested Duration
3-6 months, then as needed

Grounding Blend
Apply 2 drops to bottoms of feet in mornings. Rub a drop behind ears when anxious.

Frankincense
Put a drop under tongue. Drink water after 30 seconds.

Reassuring Blend
Apply to pulse points and temples as needed.

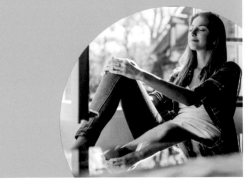

"We make a living by what we get. We make a life by what we give."

-Winston Churchill

This protocol is
brought to you by the book
Essential Oil Magic

"It's not who you are that holds you back, it's who you think you're not."

-Denis Waitley

This protocol is
brought to you by the book
Essential Oil Magic

Back, Neck, & Shoulder Pain

Description
Reduces pain and inflammation, promotes mobility.

Suggested Duration
4 weeks, then as needed

Soothing Blend
Massage in lotion into affected areas often as needed.

Polyphenol Complex
Take 1 capsule 3x/day.

Marjoram
Massage 1-2 drops into any injured muscles.

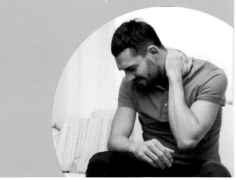

Back, Neck, & Shoulder Pain

Description
Reduces pain and inflammation, promotes mobility.

Suggested Duration
4 weeks, then as needed

Soothing Blend
Massage in lotion into affected areas often as needed.

Polyphenol Complex
Take 1 capsule 3x/day.

Marjoram
Massage 1-2 drops into any injured muscles.

"Nothing is impossible. The word
itself says *I'm possible*."

-Audrey Hepburn

This protocol is
brought to you by the book
Essential Oil Magic

"If you obey all the rules, you miss all
the fun."

-Katharine Hepburn

This protocol is
brought to you by the book
Essential Oil Magic

Colds

Description
Provides antiviral and respiratory
support.

Suggested Duration
5-10 days

Protective Blend
Drink 1-3 drops with water 3x/day.

**Protective Blend, Black Pepper, Mela-
leuca**
Rub 1-2 drops each on bottoms of feet
3x/day.

Respiratory Blend
Rub onto chest and diffuse as needed.

Vitality Supplement Trio
Take 2 of each bottle
2x/day.

Colds

Description
Provides antiviral and respiratory
support.

Suggested Duration
5-10 days

Protective Blend
Drink 1-3 drops with water 3x/day.

**Protective Blend, Black Pepper, Mela-
leuca**
Rub 1-2 drops each on bottoms of feet
3x/day.

Respiratory Blend
Rub onto chest and diffuse as needed.

Vitality Supplement Trio
Take 2 of each bottle
2x/day.

"Motivation will always beat mere talent."

-Norman Ralph Augustine

This protocol is
brought to you by the book
Essential Oil Magic

"Don't suffer from insanity, enjoy every minute of it."

-Someone wise

This protocol is
brought to you by the book
Essential Oil Magic

Depression

Description
Improves brain chemistry, supports
healthy hormone production.

Suggested Duration
3-6 months, then as needed

Joyful Blend
Carry with you, and inhale from
cupped hands often as needed for
mood support.

Frankincense or Melissa
Put a drop under the tongue 1-3x/day.

Vitality Supplement Trio
Take 2 of each bottle 2x/day.

Also consider Essential Oils + Omegas
and the Probiotic
Complex.

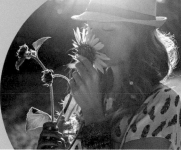

Depression

Description
Improves brain chemistry, supports
healthy hormone production.

Suggested Duration
3-6 months, then as needed

Joyful Blend
Carry with you, and inhale from
cupped hands often as needed for
mood support.

Frankincense or Melissa
Put a drop under the tongue 1-3x/day.

Vitality Supplement Trio
Take 2 of each bottle 2x/day.

Also consider Essential Oils + Omegas
and the Probiotic
Complex.

"Your imagination is your preview to
life's coming attractions."

-Albert Einstein

This protocol is
brought to you by the book
Essential Oil Magic

"Success is getting what you want.
Happiness is wanting what you get."

-Dale Carnegie

This protocol is
brought to you by the book
Essential Oil Magic

Digestive Issues

Description
Relieves inflammation, gas, and discomfort in digestive system.

Suggested Duration
2-4 weeks, then as needed

Digestive Blend
Drink 1-2 drops with water, or rub over stomach to ease discomfort.

Digestive Enzymes
Take 1 capsule w/each meal.

Probiotic Complex
Take 1 capsule w/each meal.

Frankincense & Cardamom
Rub a drop of each onto stomach reflex points in the morning.

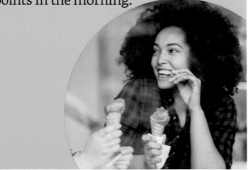

Digestive Issues

Description
Relieves inflammation, gas, and discomfort in digestive system.

Suggested Duration
2-4 weeks, then as needed

Digestive Blend
Drink 1-2 drops with water, or rub over stomach to ease discomfort.

Digestive Enzymes
Take 1 capsule w/each meal.

Probiotic Complex
Take 1 capsule w/each meal.

Frankincense & Cardamom
Rub a drop of each onto stomach reflex points in the morning.

"People often say that motivation doesn't last. Well, neither does bathing; that's why we recommend it daily."

-Zig Ziglar

This protocol is
brought to you by the book
Essential Oil Magic

"A fit, healthy body -- That is the best fashion statement."

-Jess C. Scott

This protocol is
brought to you by the book
Essential Oil Magic

Fatigue

Description
Supports adrenals, micro-circulation, and alertness.

Suggested Duration
4 weeks, then as needed

Peppermint & Rosemary
Apply 2 drops to bottoms of feet daily. Inhale from cupped hands as needed.

Lemon or Grapefruit
Use 1-3 drops in water 3x/day.

Vitality Supplement Trio
Take 2 of each bottle 2x/day.

Energy & Stamina Complex
Take 2 capsules 2x/day.

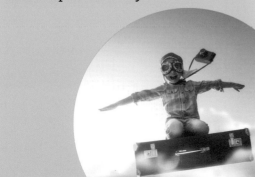

Fatigue

Description
Supports adrenals, micro-circulation, and alertness.

Suggested Duration
4 weeks, then as needed

Peppermint & Rosemary
Apply 2 drops to bottoms of feet daily. Inhale from cupped hands as needed.

Lemon or Grapefruit
Use 1-3 drops in water 3x/day.

Vitality Supplement Trio
Take 2 of each bottle 2x/day.

Energy & Stamina Complex
Take 2 capsules 2x/day.

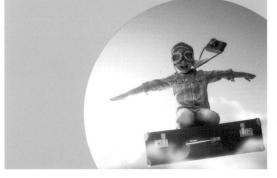

"You live only once, but if you do it right, once is enough."

-Mae West

This protocol is
brought to you by the book

"A healthy attitude is contagious, but don't wait to catch it from others; be a carrier."

-Tom Stoppard

This protocol is
brought to you by the book

Flu Bomb

Description
Combats viruses, boosts immune system, supports respiratory system.

Suggested Duration
5-10 days

Oregano, Melaleuca, Protective Blend, Lemon
Take 1-2 drops of each in a capsule 3x/day.

Digestive Blend
Drink 1-3 drops in water, or rub over stomach to ease nausea & vomiting.

Respiratory Blend
Diffuse 8 10 drops. Sit/sleep near the diffuser.

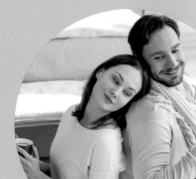

Flu Bomb

Description
Combats viruses, boosts immune system, supports respiratory system.

Suggested Duration
5-10 days

Oregano, Melaleuca, Protective Blend, Lemon
Take 1-2 drops of each in a capsule 3x/day.

Digestive Blend
Drink 1-3 drops in water, or rub over stomach to ease nausea & vomiting.

Respiratory Blend
Diffuse 8 10 drops. Sit/sleep near the diffuser.

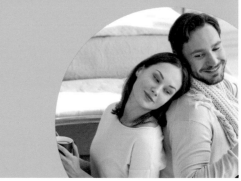

"If you're happy, if you're feeling good, then nothing else matters."

-Robin Wright

"The produce manager is more important to my children's health than the pediatrician."

-Meryl Streep

This protocol is
brought to you by the book
Essential Oil Magic

This protocol is
brought to you by the book
Essential Oil Magic